SEX BOOK

'*The Sex Book* is hugely relevant across generations and is sex education at its best. As a long-time admirer of Leeza's amazing approach to issues related to sex and relationships, for me this is a must-read compendium that takes her work to the next level.'—**Dr Nozer Sheriar, gynaecologist and obstetrician; technical advisor, South-east Asia Region, WHO; co-chair, Medical Advisory Panel, Family Planning Association of India; board member, Guttmacher Institute and Center for Catalysing Change; former secretary general, Federation of Obstetric and Gynaecological Societies of India**

'The sex book we all NEED and DESERVE! Articulate, insightful and on point.'—**Sushant Divgikr, drag icon and queer activist**

'An empowering, informative, comprehensive and delightful read! Everyone should read this book to dispel myths, understand their body better and have more pleasurable sex!'—**Dr Laurie Mintz, author of *Becoming Cliterate* and *A Tired Woman's Guide to Passionate Sex***

'*The Sex Book* is a truly wonderful encyclopaedia of sex, love, romance and pleasure that reads like having a frank conversation with a best friend. Leeza has changed the face of sex education by using the real-life concerns of her followers to bring deeply grounded advice on everything we need to know about sex but are scared to ask—from edging, emotions and ethical porn to "unknown" erogenous zones. Readers will be empowered to enjoy shame-free journeys to celebrate their sexualities, bodies and love.'—**Anne Philpott, founder, The Pleasure Project**

'Leeza answers all the questions you've been too embarrassed to ask about your body and sexual health. This book should be required reading for EVERYONE who wants to or is already having sex. Empower yourself with the knowledge found in this book and you won't regret it!'—**Dr Rena Malik, urologist and pelvic surgeon, popular medical YouTuber**

THE SEX BOOK

A JOYFUL JOURNEY OF SELF-DISCOVERY

LEEZA MANGALDAS

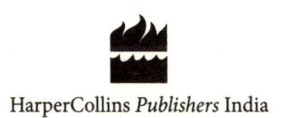

HarperCollins *Publishers* India

First published in India by HarperCollins *Publishers* 2022
4th Floor, Tower A, Building No. 10, Phase II, DLF Cyber City,
Gurugram, Haryana -122002
www.harpercollins.co.in

2 4 6 8 10 9 7 5 3 1

Copyright © Leeza Mangaldas 2022
Illustrations copyright © Ipsita Divedi 2022

P-ISBN: 978-93-5629-223-9
E-ISBN: 978-93-5629-231-4

This book is based on the knowledge and experiences of Leeza Mangaldas. The names and identifying details have been changed to protect the privacy of the individuals in this book. The views and opinions expressed in this book are the author's own and the incidents related to her personal experiences are as have been narrated by her. This book shall not, in any way, be construed as a substitute for medical advice. Neither the author, nor the publisher, is recommending any medication or treatment. Anyone struggling with issues related to sexual health should seek medical advice from a certified medical practitioner. The subject matter of this book relates strictly to imparting sex education and the infographics or diagrams are in no way lascivious or appeal to prurient interest. Any liability arising from any action undertaken by any person by relying upon any part of this book is strictly disclaimed.

Leeza Mangaldas asserts the moral right
to be identified as the author of this work.

All rights reserved. No part of this publication may be reproduced,
stored in a retrieval system, or transmitted, in any form or by any means,
electronic, mechanical, photocopying, recording or otherwise,
without the prior permission of the publishers.

Typeset in 11.5/15.7 Arno Pro at
Manipal Technologies Limited, Manipal

Printed and bound at
MicroPrints India, New Delhi

Imagine a world where all sexual experiences are consensual, safe and pleasurable.

Contents

Introduction — xvii
Glossary — xxiii

The Body: Your Genitals Are Normal — 1

The Vulva — 18

Vulva anatomy — 20

Vulva hygiene — 21

Should I get rid of my pubes? — 23

Why is the skin around the genitals darker than the rest of my body? — 25

The clitoris — 26

The G-Spot — 28

The hymen myth — 31

Does sex make the vagina loose? — 35

Vulvas and orgasms — 39

The orgasm gap — 40

Anorgasmia — 42

- Pain during sex — 42
- Vaginismus and vulvodynia — 45

Menstruation and Pregnancy — **45**

- Understanding how periods and pregnancy work — 45
- What exactly has to happen for someone to get pregnant? — 46
- Okay, so what is a period? — 48
- If you skipped a period, does it mean you're pregnant? — 49
- Period sex: Yay or nay? — 50
- Is it safe to have unprotected sex on your period? — 52
- If you have had unprotected sex, can you take a pregnancy test the same day? — 53
- PMS and PMDD — 54
- Dysmenorrhea (period pain) — 56
- PCOS — 58
- Debunking period myths — 60
- Menstrual hygiene products — 61
- Menopause — 62

Boobs — 64

- Does size matter? — 64
- Why is one boob bigger than the other? — 65
- Nipples and areola — 66
- Why do nipples get hard? — 67
- Why it's important to examine your boobs — 67

The Penis — 69

- Penis anatomy — 69
- Penis hygiene — 72
- Average penis size — 72
- Does size matter? — 73
- Curvature — 76
- Foreskin: Circumcised vs uncircumcised — 76
- Phimosis — 78
- Morning erections — 79
- Erectile dysfunction — 80
- Is masturbation bad for me and my penis? — 84

Balls: The Testes and Scrotum — 87

- The testes and scrotum — 87
- What's the difference between sperm and semen? — 88

What is precum?	90
Can you get pregnant from precum?	90
Nightfall	91
Premature ejaculation	92
What is the refractory period?	94
'Blue balls'	95
Delayed ejaculation	96

The Prostate — **97**

An erogenous zone many don't know about!	97

Gender-affirming Surgery and the Genitals — **98**

What is gender-affirming surgery?	98
What is a neopenis and a neovagina?	98
What is gender dysphoria?	99

Sex : What You Need to Know Long Before You Get Naked — 103

First Sexual Experiences — **105**

What is the 'right' age to have sex?	105
What is sex like the first time?	108

Consent — **113**

What is consent?	113

Does asking for consent 'kill the mood'? ... 117
Consent matters, no matter your gender ... 120
Consent as a daily practice ... 121
Consent 101: What everyone should know ... 122

Safer Sex: Protection and Contraception ... **124**

What methods protect against both
STIs and pregnancy? ... 124

Regular condoms ... 125

Internal condoms ... 126

Dental dams ... 127

Condom FAQs ... 128

Contraception: Birth control methods
beyond condoms ... 133

The Copper-T ... 135

Oral contraceptive pills ... 137

Hormonal IUDs ... 139

What's the difference between birth
control pills, emergency contraception and
abortion pills? ... 142

Understanding Abortion in India ... **144**

Is abortion legal in India? ... 145

Can you get an abortion if you are not married? 147

Can you get an abortion if you are under the age of eighteen? 147

How safe is abortion? 148

What sort of procedures does a safe abortion entail? 148

Are abortions painful? 149

How common is abortion? 149

Why is it important that we support the right to choose? 150

Emotional Safety **151**

Understanding 'aftercare' 151

Why do people sometimes cry after sex? 153

Pleasure: Everyone Deserves It! 155

Self-pleasure 159

A gateway to sexual self-knowledge 159

I've never masturbated. How do I go about it? 164

Is it okay to masturbate if I'm in a relationship? 166

What is mutual masturbation? 167

Contents   xiii

Orgasms   **169**

What is an orgasm and how do I know if I've had one?   169

Foreplay   **172**

What is foreplay?   172

Kissing   **173**

How to be a 'good kisser'   173

Fingering and Hand Jobs   **175**

How can I use my hands to provide pleasure?   175

Oral Sex   **177**

How do you have oral sex safely?   179

Is it okay to swallow semen and vaginal fluids?   179

Is it better to spit or swallow when giving a blowjob?   180

Should I worry about how I taste and smell down there?   180

Do I have to wax or shave my pubic hair if I want to receive oral sex?   181

How do I initiate oral sex?   182

How do I get good at oral sex?   183

How to lick a pussy   184

Vaginal Sex — 186

Why do many women and vulva-owners find it difficult to orgasm during intercourse? — 186

How to have an orgasm for people with vulvas — 186

How can penetrative intercourse become more pleasurable for vulva-owners? — 187

Positions to try — 189

What is squirting? — 191

How can I last longer in bed? — 192

What is edging? — 193

Anal Sex — 193

Butt stuff: What do I need to know? — 193

The importance of condoms and lube — 194

Will there be poop? — 194

Anal fingering — 194

Rimming — 195

Anal sex — 196

Pegging — 198

Arousal — 199

What's the most powerful sexual organ? — 199

Arousal non-concordance 201
Moaning 203
Dirty talk 206

Lube **208**
What is lube? 208
Which lube should you use? 210

Sex Toys **212**
What are sex toys? 212
Types of sex toys 214
How to choose a sex toy 215

Fantasies **220**
Common sexual fantasies 220
What is roleplay? 221

Fetishes and Kinks **221**
What is a fetish? 221
What is a kink? 222
Common kinks and fetishes 223

Porn **227**
Is porn helpful or harmful? 227
What is ethical porn? 229

Is porn addiction real? 231

What shapes our sexual and
romantic aspirations? 234

Relationships: Navigating Sexuality Together 237

Talking to your parents/kids/family
about sex 239

What does a healthy relationship look like? 246

How important is sex to a relationship? 247

Toxic masculinity 250

Non-monogamy 253

Confused about your sexuality? 255

Love 257

Afterword 260

Further reading 263

Acknowledgements 265

About the Author 267

Introduction

As human beings, we've been trying to make sense of ourselves—our lives, our sexualities, our bodies, our desires, our identities—for centuries. And we like simple answers: Yes/No, Good/Bad, Right/Wrong. Male or Female; Queer or Straight; Virgin or Whore; Clean or Dirty; Desirable or Disgusting.

But the truth is, our lives and our bodies, and our identities, are nuanced and complex. Being human and, moreover, being sexual—is not a neat and tidy experience. It's complicated, varied, and confusing. And that's okay! Simply accepting this fact is where we've got to start. There is no single 'right' way to be a human, there is no one 'ideal' body and there is no 'correct' way to have sex. That's what makes the human experience inexplicably profound and wonderful.

As someone who has created sex-positive conversations online for over half a decade, and as one of the first people to do so on social media in India, my inboxes are flooded with messages from people of all genders and ages, from all over the country and even the world. And if I were to deconstruct the questions I receive into one overarching concern, what I get asked over and over and over again is essentially this: 'Am I normal?'

From conversations with other sex educators in India, as well as from places as varied as Kenya and Canada, I know that this holds true for most of us, no matter where we are based. From questions about penis size or boob size to concerns about 'performance', from questions about fantasies to questions about sexual orientation; whether it's sexual health or pleasure—people simply want to be reassured that there's nothing *wrong* with them—their bodies, their curiosities, their desires.

Here's why we all have this fear. The world is still pretty damn sex-negative globally. (Thanks to patriarchy, religion, colonialism and multiple other cultural and societal forces that have sought to surveil and control people's sexual and reproductive choices for centuries.) So most of us have inherited a ton of shame and fear and guilt when it comes to how we think about sex and the body.

Consider the fact that many parents still teach their toddlers that the preferred euphemism for their genitals is 'shame shame'. Consider the fact that the Latin word for external genitals, particularly those of a woman—still sometimes used in medical and scientific contexts—is *pudendum*, which has its etymological origins in the word *pudere,* which literally means 'to be ashamed'. Consider the biblical stories of Adam and Eve, the Original *Sin*; and of the *Virgin* Mary, and how the arising moral framework that values sexual 'purity' (particularly of women) and posits sex as 'sinful' was disseminated throughout the world via colonialism.

It's important to consider the stories we've been told for centuries and how they've shaped our attitudes and beliefs so that we can unpack the shame and carefully select what we want to keep and what we want to let go of.

Here's what most of us come into adulthood at least somewhat believing about sex:

Sex, in general, is dangerous, immoral, shameful, sinful. Globally, sex is still presented as truly 'respectable' only in the context of heterosexual marriage. Sex between a man and a woman, after marriage, and ideally with the primary intent to have a child, lies at the pinnacle of 'acceptability', with everything else falling short. In India, and in many other parts of the world too, this ought to be a same-religion, same-caste marriage, so that existing social hierarchies can literally be reproduced. The woman should be a virgin, because in a patriarchal society, a woman's sexual 'chastity' is a mark of her and her family's 'honour' to be preserved by her father till she is married, after which she becomes the property of her husband.

We're told anything outside of this incredibly oppressive and narrow framework—such as premarital sex, particularly unmarried women having sex, queer sex, paid sex, sex with more than one partner, and even masturbation—is bad, dirty, dishonourable, *punishable*. And we're discouraged from even talking about sex, let alone questioning these beliefs, because, well, *log kya kahenge? What will people say?*

The combination of the societal shame and stigma along with the ensuing lack of accurate information about sex, sexual health and the body, means that most people are worried that there's something *very* wrong with them when it comes to their sexual selves. Because if we're being honest, our lived experiences do not tidily fit into that rigid and oppressive narrative. Far from it.

And so, as we enter adulthood, we often pathologize our own (very normal) bodies and desires, because even thinking a sexual thought or seeking to access contraception can seem transgressive—forget about delving into questions about our sexual orientation or exploring how our body works in relation to pleasure.

This refusal to talk about sex—at home, in school, in our communities—at best results in generations of clueless young people left to figure out everything for themselves, from how to have safe sex to how to have an orgasm; but at worst, it results in things like women being killed for not bleeding on their wedding night, and queer teens being sent to quacks to be 'cured' by conversion therapy.

Comprehensive Sex Education that is pleasure-inclusive and queer-inclusive is central to greater gender equality, to improved sexual and reproductive health and rights, to ending sexual- and gender-based violence, and to achieving a safer, kinder, more joyful world.

And while some people mistakenly think that access to sex education will result in everyone having more sex at a younger age, in fact, studies globally have shown that people who *can* talk to a parent, teacher or caregiver about sex are more likely to delay having sex and less likely to make choices that put their own or another's health and safety at risk.

Now, we could wait around and hope for the day when schools all over the world have comprehensive Sex Ed programmes, but we'd be waiting for a long time. So how about we proactively seek out factful, judgment-free information ourselves and at least within our own homes, relationships and communities, begin to normalize talking about this stuff.

As a young, unmarried Indian woman trying to navigate my own sexuality, sexual health and relationships, I found there to be a huge lack of easily accessible and culturally relevant information and resources about sex. Where could one go for scientifically accurate and shame-free conversations about this important aspect of our lives? This was what inspired me to start my digital sex-education platforms. And with this book, I hope to make it even easier to access all the information I've been trying to share, because now it's all in one place.

I hope together we can eliminate our shame and fill some of the gaps in our knowledge so that we are equipped to make better, safer, more informed, more empathetic and more pleasurable choices in our sexual lives.

*Please note: **Whenever I've quoted questions or messages from my viewers, names have been changed to protect their privacy.**

Glossary

Now that you've decided to think about sexuality and identity, here's a list of terms that will be useful to understand.

It's impossible to talk about sex without also wrapping our heads around sexuality, gender, sexual orientation—and identity at large. And each of these concepts also has its own subsets of related ideas that are important to know. So here's a list of terms that I hope you will read through carefully rather than skip over. That's the whole point of this book for me—unlike in an Instagram reel, I have more than 90 seconds of your time here to make my points!

Sex

Depending on context, 'sex' typically refers to either penetrative sexual intercourse or to biological sex/sex assigned at birth—the classification of individuals into two major groups: Male and Female, on the basis of the anatomy of their genitals and reproductive organs. However, both these traditional definitions of the word sex require expansion—because sex is in fact more than just penis-in-vagina penetration, and 'biological' sex is more complicated and variable than a rigid, binary only-either-M-or-F-approach allows room for.

Sexual Orientation

One's sexual orientation is shaped by who one is sexually attracted to and/or whether one feels sexual attraction or desire. Some people do not experience sexual desire at all, and that's normal too.

Straight (also called heterosexual, meaning attraction to the opposite sex), Gay (also called homosexual, meaning attraction to the same sex, and most often used to describe men who are attracted to men), Lesbian (women who are attracted to women), Bisexual (people attracted to more than one gender), Pansexual (people attracted to all genders, or attracted to people regardless of gender), Asexual (people who are not driven by sexual attraction)—are a few examples of sexual orientations.

However, these labels are intended to help you describe how you experience attraction, not make you feel boxed in. If using a label helps you navigate and affirm your own identity, great! If you prefer not to use a label, or you find that a label that once resonated with you no longer does, that's fine too! We deserve to be able to communicate about our sexuality in the ways that feel truest to us.

We grow up thinking that heterosexuality—opposite-sex desire—men being attracted to women and women being attracted to men—is the default or 'normal' orientation. And this is part of the conditioning of the heteronormative, patriarchal system we're all a little bit trapped in. But, in fact, historically, many cultures including our own have long acknowledged and celebrated a far more fluid view of human desire.

A combination of biological, psychological, social and cultural factors may influence how you experience desire and who you're attracted to, and over time you may discover aspects of your own sexuality that you hadn't acknowledged before. Some people experience their sexual orientation as 'I was born this way'—it's something innate, something they've always known. But for others, it can be a process of self-discovery over time.

Sexuality

Sexuality isn't exactly the same as sex or sexual orientation. Although your sexual experiences and sexual orientation are likely to shape and be shaped by your sexuality.

Sexuality has to do with your identity and humanness, how you experience the world, and how you experience your body, your desires and your relationships.

It can encompass much of your physical, emotional, social, and even spiritual, feelings and behaviours, and is often informed by your cultural context. We all deserve to be able to explore and understand our sexuality safely and without shame.

Your sexuality becomes a part of who you are, how you see yourself, how you express yourself, and how others see you. It too may evolve over time as your circumstances evolve and you get to know yourself better.

Gender

While gender is still often imperfectly used as a synonym for sex assigned at birth, gender, in fact, refers to the behavioural, cultural or psychological characteristics associated with ideas of 'masculinity' and 'femininity'.

Gender identity can be understood as one's own perception of one's identity in relation to social constructs around gender. One's gender identity need not necessarily correspond with what genitals one has, and this is important to understand.

When a doctor assigns a baby either 'Male' or 'Female' at birth, based on whether the baby's genitals more closely resemble a penis or a vulva, this act of assignment too often carries the implicit expectation that future gender identity ought to develop in alignment with the sex assigned.

It is important to understand that gender roles are socially, rather than biologically, constructed. From birth, society places very different conditionings and expectations on 'Boys' and 'Girls', 'Men' and 'Women'—such as, 'blue is for boys, pink is for girls'; 'girls ought to take an interest in their appearance, boys ought to play sport'; 'boys shouldn't cry, girls shouldn't sit with their legs apart'; 'men must accrue wealth and property, women must tend to the home and the children'.

These restrictive gender expectations have been so pervasive that for centuries we've been prescribed a very narrow code of acceptable behaviours, careers, dressing and appearance, and even what it's okay to say, where it's okay to go and who it's okay to love, based on whether we are 'men' or 'women'. And the resulting social inequalities and oppression have been wrongly passed off as if they're simply the 'natural' order of things.

Even desirability and attractiveness are often couched in stringent definitions by our society as if they are correlated to how 'masculine' a man is (eg. muscular, tall, bearded, strong, aggressive) and how 'feminine' a woman is (eg. big breasts, small waist, long hair, docile, pleasant), so much so that to call a girl 'manly' or to call a man 'girly' is to be perceived as an insult. Thankfully we're finally starting to see how absurd all of this is.

Gender, like 'biological' sex, has long been constructed in the context of a colonial, patriarchal society and via a binary lens, and so its constructs have not only historically upheld 'male' traits as superior to 'female' traits, valuing men at the cost of women (sexism, misogyny), it has also restricted the self-expression of 'men' and 'women' (toxic masculinity, compulsory femininity) and neglected to accommodate people whose gender identity does not conform to the categories of either 'man' or 'woman'.

As queer, trans and non-binary experiences finally begin to receive long overdue public and media representation, the ways we think about gender are also undergoing a radical re-examination. Instead of thinking of gender as if it is strictly biologically determined, it is important to reflect on one's own personal sense or conception of one's gender.

Your gender identity is how *you* identify yourself, and how you'd like to be seen and understood by the world. It could be in accordance with, in opposition to, or outside of the gender binary and/or your sex assigned at birth. It is the gender identity that feels truest to your own experiences, emotions and self-perception.

Just as 'man' and 'woman' are valid gender identities, so also 'non-binary', 'gender fluid', 'gender non-conforming', 'gender queer' are equally valid identities.

In an ideal world where gender isn't used as a tool of oppression and control, your gender identity would always be yours to determine and express, and no one else's business but your own.

Cis

Cis is short for cisgender. A cis person is someone whose gender identity 'corresponds' with the sex they were assigned at birth.

Trans

Trans is short for transgender. It is an umbrella term to describe people whose gender identity does not correspond with the sex they were assigned at birth. People for whom the gender binary itself simply holds no resonance may also identify as trans.

Some trans people may choose to have hormone therapy and/or surgery to affirm their gender identity. However, an individual does not have to have gender-affirming hormone therapy or surgery in order to identify as trans.

In the words of Stevie Lang (@_steviewrites on Instagram), whose writing on gender and identity I greatly admire, trans identity powerfully illuminates the fact that we as human beings 'should be free to transcend the categories and stereotypes of gender that were placed on us at birth', such that gender, instead of being something that traps us with its demands and expectations, can instead become a 'site of liberation and joy'.

Non-Binary

A 'binary' is something with two parts, often defined in opposition to each other. The prevalent idea that there are only two genders—'man' and 'woman'—is called the 'gender binary'.

While many people do identify as either men or women, gender identity exists beyond the binary. Some people identify as neither man nor woman. Some people may identify as both masculine and feminine, while others don't identify with any gender. Some people may identify with a gender for a time and then discover new aspects of their gender identity. Non-binary, genderqueer, gender non-conforming, gender fluid and agender are some umbrella terms for identities that transcend the confines of the 'gender binary'.

Asexuality

Ironically, even though society judges and shames people for having sex, it also shames and invisibilizes asexual identity. Asexuality is a sexual orientation. Some people are not driven by sex, and/or may have no desire for sex. Just like other sexual orientations, being asexual is not a 'condition' that needs to be 'fixed'. And there isn't a single, monolithic way to be asexual. It can be helpful to think of asexuality as a spectrum. Some asexual folks or 'aces' may seek romantic relationships and experience romantic desire but have no interest in sex; some seek neither romantic nor sexual relationships; and some may choose to have sex with their partner—there isn't a single 'right' way to be asexual, just as there isn't a single 'right' way to be any identity.

Queer

Queer is an umbrella term that encompasses all identities that resist the heteronormative relationship scripts and/or rigidly binary gender norms that society enforces. Initially, 'queer' was a homophobic, transphobic slur. However, the word has been reclaimed, and encompasses the spectrum of sexual orientations and gender identities that exist beyond just heterosexual and/

or cisgender. Some people interrogating heteronormativity and/or the gender binary to better understand their own identity may also simply identify with the broader term 'queer' rather than a more specific sexual orientation label or gender identity label.

Patriarchy

Patriarchy is the still globally prevalent gendered ordering system around which society, religion, governance, and therefore pretty much every other aspect of everyday life, has been and largely continues to be structured around, of which the foundational assumptions are that gender is binary, that male superiority is a 'fact of nature', and that women are the property of men and exist primarily to bear them children—ideally male heirs.

Patriarchal societies have long been obsessed with paternity—i.e. they operate on the premise that the man ought to be the head of the family and to make sure that the man who thinks he is the father is indeed the father of his son—women's bodies and sexual agency must be entirely controlled and surveilled, and a family's honour must be linked to the chastity of its women. A woman is to be her father's property until marriage, after which she becomes her husband's property, and she is to bear a male heir. All this might sound rather like it belongs in the Stone Age, but when you really think about it, it's still how much of the world functions.

In patriarchal societies, a woman's worth is thus defined by her sexual inexperience, yet, paradoxically, also by her willingness to have children, while a man's worth is defined by his proximity to wealth and property. And too often, anyone who does not conform to the gender binary and to a heteronormative relationship structure is an 'aberration' and must be punished.

Marriage is the cornerstone of patriarchy. For centuries, globally, marriage was restricted to only heterosexual, endogamous alliances (endogamy refers to the custom of marrying only within one's own community) so that social hierarchies could literally be reproduced. Even today, in India, same-sex marriage is illegal, and the vast majority of people have no choice but to enter into a heterosexual marriage with a partner from the same religion, caste and community, and have a child.

Once you start to understand what patriarchy is, you'll start to see its talons everywhere. It is so ubiquitous and generationally ingrained in us that, at first, it may be hard to see. But once you see it, you can't unsee it. Patriarchy benefits no one, not even men.

Casteism

Casteism is systemic and interpersonal discrimination on the basis of caste. It is important that we think about casteism in relation to sexuality and relationships because, in many ways, our personal lives continue to uphold casteism, given the social emphasis on endogamy. Marriage remains a staunchly casteist institution in India, and even though inter-caste marriage is legal, an incredibly small fraction of the total number of marriages that take place in the country each year are inter-caste, and an even smaller fraction are between people of oppressor castes and those oppressed. By choosing, or being coerced, to date and marry only within our own caste, we literally end up reproducing caste hierarchies. Just as much as we need to interrogate the ways our experiences of gender, sexuality and the body are coloured by oppression and exclusion, we also need to think about how the attitudes and practices we participate in may perpetuate oppression and exclusion.

Ableism

Ableism is systemic and interpersonal discrimination against people with disabilities. Ableism is the tendency to view the world from an able-bodied lens, ignoring or disregarding the needs and experiences of people with disabilities. Ableism often makes itself felt as an unexamined bias that pits non-disabled people as the 'standard' and disabled folks as 'less-than', the fact that making physical spaces, services and resources accessible to people with disabilities still largely remains an afterthought, as well as harmful stereotypes, misconceptions and generalizations around people with disabilities. A lot of existing notions around sex, sexuality, sexual health, pleasure, desire and the body are inherently ableist and require re-examination.

Privilege

Privilege refers to the advantage or position of power that certain people or groups of people have over others. In society globally, the list of those who are privileged is long. For example, white people, men, upper-class, oppressor-caste, cis and heterosexual people, the able-bodied and those who belong to a country's dominant religious group enjoy certain privileges, as compared to people of colour, working-class, oppressed caste, trans and queer people, people with disabilities, and those who belong to religious minorities.

It is important to think about the privileges one has, as well as the systemic oppressions one faces, as various forms of privilege and oppression intersect and overlap in ways that need to be examined critically.

For example, I am a brown woman, but I am also cis, able- bodied, upper class and upper caste. As a woman and a person of colour, I am constantly thinking about the ways in which my freedom and identity have been systematically targeted throughout history and well into the present day by a white-supremacist, patriarchal global society. But I must also consider the ways in which the positions of privilege I simultaneously occupy have contributed to the oppression of others. Dismantling oppression is the dismantling of all types of oppression.

Internalized Oppression

When a group has been treated as subordinate and inferior to another group for so long and so relentlessly that its members may start to see themselves as inherently inferior to the privileged group, thereby further perpetuating their own oppression.

For example, while it would seem that only men could be misogynists, only white people could be racist, only straight people could be homophobic, only cis people could be transphobic, or only thin people could fat-shame, the oppression and prejudice against these affected groups have been so pervasive that even women can internalize misogyny, a dark-skinned person can internalize colourism, a gay person can internalize homophobia, a trans person can internalize transphobia, a fat person can internalize fat phobia, and so on. These are just a few examples—internalized oppression can occur as a result of all forms of systemic oppression.

The Body

Your Genitals Are Normal

I had my first sexual experience in the winter of my freshman year in college. I was dating a really sweet guy, my first real 'boyfriend'. A few months into the relationship, we decided we were ready to 'do it'.

We wanted 'it' to be special, so we made a reservation at a nice restaurant for dinner that weekend, and the plan was to then come back to my dorm room, light candles and play soft music, get naked, and see where things go. We bought condoms, fresh strawberries and a can of whipped cream—all in anticipation of our upcoming adventure.

Dinner was entirely lovely and romantic, and back at my dorm room, after we'd been kissing and cuddling for a while, I decided it was time to get up close and personal with his penis, so I sidled halfway down the bed and began undoing his pants.

But when I found my actual face a few inches away from an actual penis and scrotum, I was woefully ill-equipped to make sense of what I saw.

Coming into that experience, I knew *so little* about what real genitals look like. Mine is probably the last generation to have grown up without smartphones. I had never watched porn. This was the first time I was seeing an actual penis. And I was expecting to see two testicles, but I could see only one.

I'd only ever seen drawings of penises like the sort people would make on the chalkboard when the teacher wasn't looking: two circles and a long oval. Even the diagrams in the chapter on the reproductive system in Bio class—I was a total nerd and could label them perfectly—didn't prepare me for what real balls actually looked like.

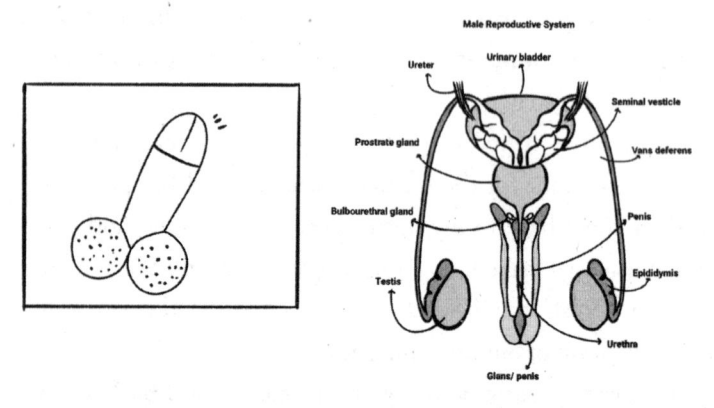

I was expecting there'd be two separate spheres under his penis, not two spheres in one bag that can almost seem like one large blobby sphere.

I tried my best to keep a straight face, but my head was a muddle of confusion and curiosity.

(Younger me was much less aware of genital diversity, and even less so of the notion that if he did have only one ball, it's not a big deal.)

Not wanting to embarrass him, or myself, I closed my eyes and placed my hands on his penis, and as I felt around, it dawned on me.

'Ohhhh he does have two balls—they're both just packed into one sac! OHHHHH!!!!'

That's how eighteen-year-old me learned about the scrotum.

So I can empathize with the thousands of questions and concerns I receive from people worried about whether their genitals are normal. Here is just a small sampling:

'My penis is small and a little curved, should I be worried?'

'I think one of my testicles is slightly bigger than the other, am I a freak?'

'My clitoris is tiny and hard to find, totally hidden under the hood, is something wrong with me?'

'My inner labia dangles and protrudes outward, it looks nothing like the lady bits I've seen in porn.'

'My foreskin droops over the top of my penis when I'm not erect. I'm afraid it looks weird.'

Our genitals are as diverse as our faces. Since we get to see hundreds of thousands of faces over the course of our lives, we know that facial features can take all kinds of shapes and colours and textures and combinations. We don't see people's genitals nearly as often. And many of us, particularly people with vulvas, may never even have taken a close look at our own. There's actually a lot of variation in terms of how external genitalia can look—there is no single right colour, size or shape. Everyone has their own unique features.

Perhaps internet porn has now changed that in some ways—we have easier access than ever before to imagery of sex and genitalia. But most mainstream porn performers are white, and many have had plastic surgery, pubic hair removal, anal bleaching, and other such procedures—after all, in many cases, their income depends on how closely their bodies conform to the archetypal porn aesthetic.

Fortunately, there are now more independent adult filmmakers prioritizing an authentic representation of diverse identities, sexualities and body types, in 'ethical', 'feminist', 'indie' porn. But most of the performers in mainstream big-studio-produced porn still likely either fit a rather narrow 'pornstar' archetype, or are fetishized for looking a certain way if they don't.

In the absence of comprehensive sex education in schools, and a reticence around talking about sex at home, young people either have no really accurate reference points for understanding sex and the genitals as they come into their own first sexual experiences (like the younger me), or—and this is much more likely, given the ubiquity of smartphones and the internet now—it's the free, mainstream internet porn where men have huge penises and women have huge breasts and hairless vulvas and men can go on for hours and the acts are often overwhelmingly violent and misogynistic—that becomes the inevitable first visual reference point.

In high school biology lessons (if your school didn't skip the chapter altogether), we are taught about sex only in the context of reproduction. We may see a diagram of the insides of a penis and the testes perhaps, and we may see the uterus and the ovaries perhaps, and if we are lucky, we may even see a little canal labelled the vagina, but we rarely see properly labelled diagrams of the external genitals, particularly the vulva (or the scrotum, for that matter!) And we certainly never even hear about the clitoris.

The Body 7

If we did get taught the chapter, we're likely to have seen a diagram like this:

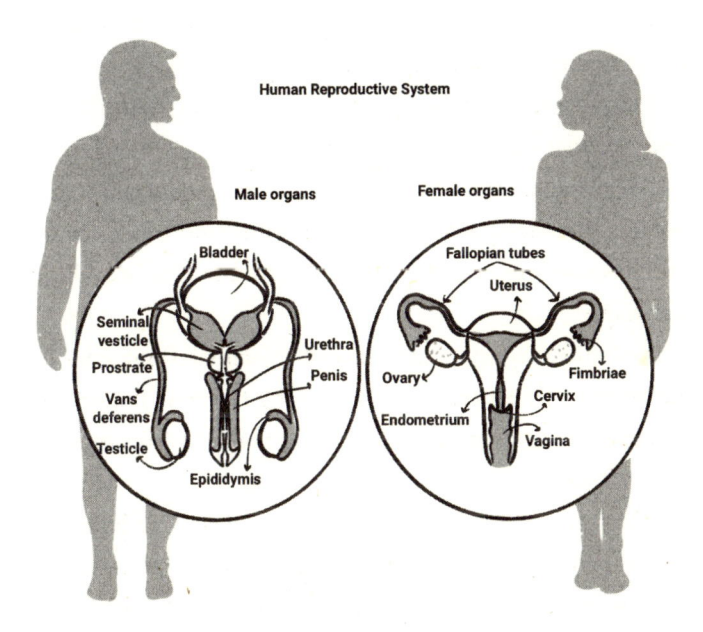

Human Reproductive System

Male organs — Bladder, Seminal vesicle, Prostrate, Vans deferens, Testicle, Urethra, Penis, Epididymis

Female organs — Fallopian tubes, Uterus, Ovary, Endometrium, Fimbriae, Cervix, Vagina

As a result, most of us think that men have a penis (and if you're like me, two SEPARATE balls—I mean, just look at how far away they seem in this diagram—can you blame me for not realizing they're both in the same sac?) and that women have vaginas, and the 'female' equivalent of the 'male' penis is the vagina, and that sex equals penis-in-vagina.

But this is a highly oversimplified portrayal of gender, the genitals and sex.

Neither mainstream porn nor the reproductive system lesson in most schools tells you what you need to know about sex and the body, health and pleasure and identity, in a way that makes this stuff feel normal, comfortable, easy to understand, safe and worthy of exploration.

We're constantly told about *men* and *women* and *male* and *female* bodies as if they're totally disparate categories. But get this: as foetuses, *we all start off exactly the same, with the exact same genital tissue.*

We all begin with a little genital tubercle and a labioscrotal swelling that then goes on to become either more like a clitoris and vulva or more like a penis and scrotum as we develop in the womb.

As Emily Nagoski, internationally celebrated sex educator and author of the ground-breaking book *Come As You Are* likes to say: 'We are all made of the same parts, just organized in different ways.'

Thus, regardless of what our sex assigned at birth may be, our genitals are similar in so many ways. Both the clitoris and the penis have a head (glans) and a shaft; just as the clitoris has the clitoral hood, the penis has a foreskin; both the clitoris and the penis become engorged with blood when aroused; and stimulation of the penis and the clitoris are both central to sexual pleasure. Likewise, the skin of the labial folds on a vulva and the skin of the scrotum or ball sac also feel remarkably alike.

Also, while for most people, the eventual sexual differentiation of the foetus means that you are born with either penis and testes or vulva and ovaries, it is estimated that at least 1.7 per cent of the global population are born intersex

Sexual Differentiation: External Genetalia

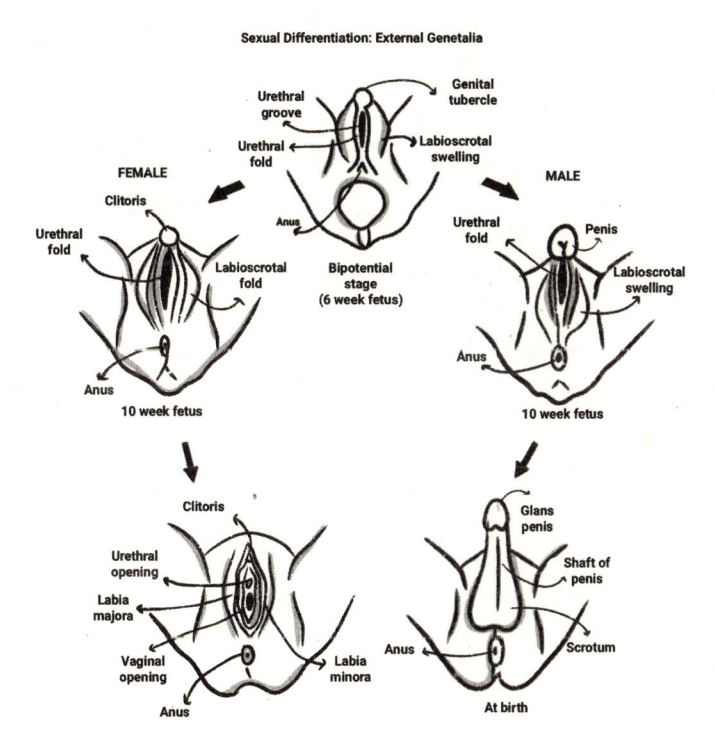

We all start off the same

(relating to or denoting a person that has both 'male' and 'female' biological traits).[1]

---

1. 'The Way We Think About Biological Sex Is Wrong', Emily Quinn, Ted.com, November 2018, https://www.ted.com/talks/emily_quinn_the_way_we_think_about_biological_sex_is_wrong?language=en. Accessed 24 March 2021.

Similarities between the Penis and the Clitoris

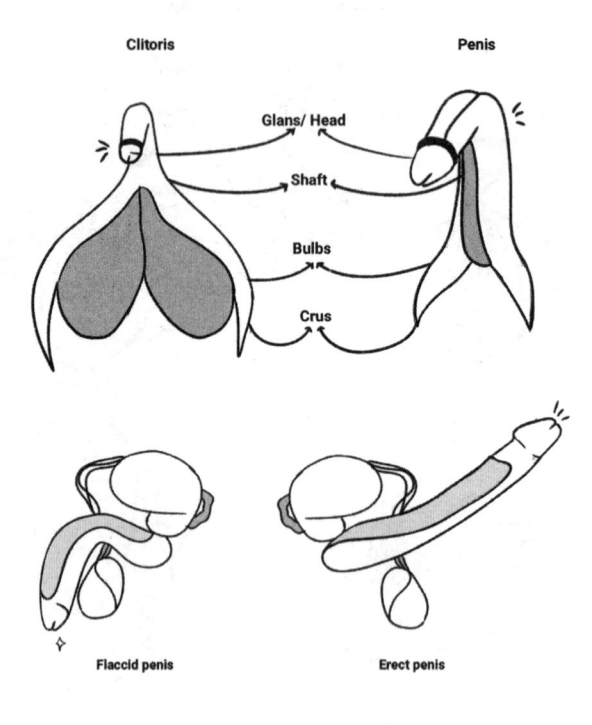

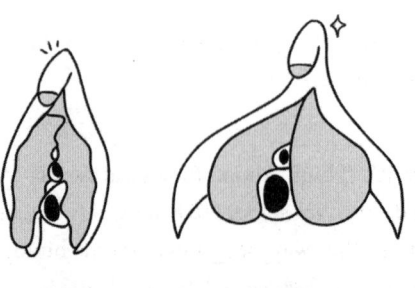

Clitoris — Penis

- Glans/ Head
- Shaft
- Bulbs
- Crus

Flaccid penis

Erect penis

Flaccid clitoris

Erect clitoris

The comparison that's often drawn to help people make sense of that statistic is that there are at least as many intersex people as there are redheads, or people with green eyes, in the world.

An intersex individual's chromosomes, external genitals, internal reproductive organs, and hormone levels, may have certain traits typically considered 'male', and other traits typically considered 'female'.

Unfortunately, instead of simply assigning babies whose bodies do not conform exactly to typically 'male' or typically 'female' traits as intersex, many doctors try to assign intersex infants as either male or female, and then recommend surgeries and procedures to 'normalize' their bodies such that their genitals and secondary sex characteristics correspond more with the sex assigned—even when the person's existing anatomy poses no health complications. In these ways, intersex identity has been both stigmatized, as well as invisiblized.

Actually, most of us don't even know very much about our genitals. Most of us haven't ever taken a long, close look at these beautiful and intimate parts of our own bodies. Many people with vulvas don't know that the clitoris extends internally too; many people with penises don't know what or where their

---

I highly recommend watching intersex activist and artist Emily Quinn's fantastic TED Talk on the subject if you're interested in hearing a first-hand perspective of what it means to be intersex and why our existing binary frameworks within which we learn about sex and gender are inadequate.

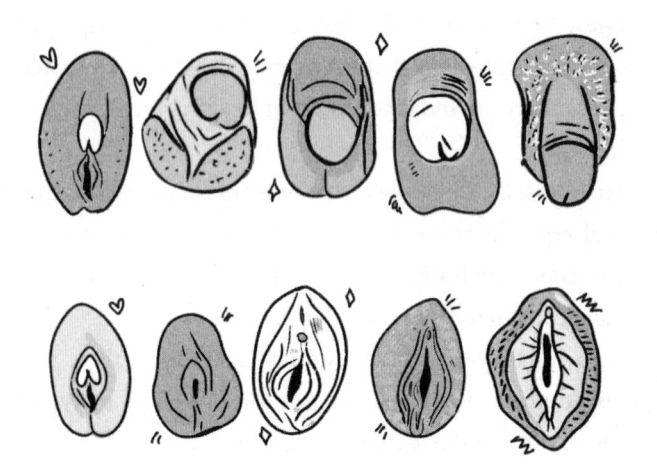

Genitals come in all shapes and sizes. Genital diversity is normal!

prostate is. And yet, given how rigidly our society is structured around a binary categorization of sex and gender, our genitals as perceived by the doctor when we were born go on to dictate much of the course of the rest of our lives.

M or F?

What you are assigned based on your genitals at birth, and how closely you are able to conform to the socially constructed gender expectations attached to this binary categorization of sex, still goes on to determine what opportunities are within the realm of possibility or acceptability for you to access or even aspire to. The schools we go to, the jobs we choose, the clothes we wear, the things we say, the places we can visit, who we are allowed to love, who we get to be in this world—these are so often dictated to us on the basis of whether we have a penis or a vulva. What an oppressive and limiting framework within which to exist.

But this rigidly binary approach is so much a part of the fabric of patriarchal society that many of us never question it. In fact, many of us staunchly hold on to and defend it, even though it cages us all.

This rigid gender binary is reiterated even via seemingly innocuous everyday choices we have to make—which public restroom to use, which queue to stand in, which box to tick on a form—that we must be either male or female, men or women, boys or girls. Even things that ostensibly have nothing to do with sex or gender—what we eat, what bath products we use or even the books we read—are often sold to us as if they are necessarily different.

But simply because I have a vagina, must I necessarily like pink, play with dolls, wear dresses, have long hair, sit with my legs crossed, be quiet and likeable, learn to cook, aspire for marriage, and become a mother? Simply because you have a penis, must you like blue, play sports, wear pants, have short hair, be strong and aggressive, hide your emotions, and dedicate your life to acquiring money and property? Why must we continue to define ideals of femininity and masculinity in these narrow and stereotypical ways?

Dismantling the gender binary can seem like a radical idea, given the global pervasiveness of a patriarchal, cis heteronormative social framework. But it is worth remembering that, historically, several cultures—including our own—accommodated for a more fluid view.

The binary framework of 'biological sex' that many of us assume to be the 'natural' categorization of 'male' and 'female' is, in fact, a framework that was created by white male scientists in the nineteenth century, much the same way they tried to create a hierarchy among races: all in order to justify discrimination against women, indigenous people and people of colour.

Socially constructed ideas of gender have tried to impose an oppressive mesh of what is 'appropriate' and 'natural' when it comes to the appearances and behaviours of 'men' and 'women', falsely using 'biology' as a basis for justification.

In contrast to gender binarism, the Bugis people, an ethnic group in Indonesia, have for centuries recognized a multiplicity of genders, and anthropologists have suggested similar traditions existed in Thailand and Malaysia. Native Hawaiians and Tahitians as well as some Native Americans have also traditionally conceptualized gender in a fluid rather than binary way, with multiple gender categories.

India and other South Asian cultures too have long recognized that gender identity exists beyond the binary, and allude to the idea that the masculine and the feminine are connected, rather than opposed, even in the representation of Hindu deities such as Ardhanarishvara—Shiva and Parvati in a beautiful composite form.

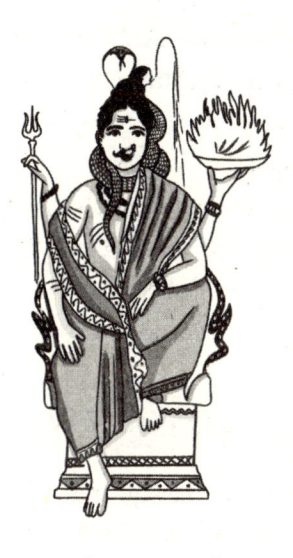

If we let go of our attachment to a binary conception of sex and gender and, instead, adopt a more inclusive framework to think about gender, sex and sexuality as a constellation of wonderful, varied and equally valid possibilities of human identity, we'd be able to acknowledge and appreciate the entire range and complexity of variations—and similarities—across our bodies, our identities and our preferences—instead of forcing ourselves, and each other, into boxes we don't necessarily fit into.

'People with penises' and **'people with vulvas'** are terms used in order not to conflate gender with genitals, and these are the terms I'm going to be using in this book instead of only saying 'men' and 'women' or 'male' and 'female' when speaking in general objective terms about the genitals and the body.

When I do use the terms 'men' and 'women', it is with regard to how those gender identities condition certain social and bodily experiences, as opposed to as indicators or descriptors of anatomy in general.

No matter what our bodies look like, we get to decide what identity labels affirm our sense of self, and we also have the freedom to choose none at all.

Oh, and your genitals are normal. I promise.

> ## GO FOLLOW
>
> If you're interested in thinking more about where ideas around sex and gender come from, and what they mean, I highly recommend following gender non-conforming author, artist, speaker and activist, **Alok Vaid-Menon,** on Instagram (@alokvmenon) as well as reading their book, *Beyond the Gender Binary*. In addition to their exquisite images, writing and poetry, they also share superb book reports via which I have discovered some of the most eye-opening writing about the history and implications of the sex and gender binaries. Here are three books I especially enjoyed: *Myths of Gender: Biological Theories about Women and Men* by Anne Fausto-Sterling, *Brain Storm: The Flaws in the Science of Sex Differences* by Rebecca M. Jordan-Young and *Sexual Science: The Victorian Construction of Womanhood* by Cynthia Eagle Russett.

> And for wonderfully informative diagrams and educational information about genital anatomy, check out @vielma.art. Stefanie Grübl is an artist and sexuality educator based in Austria who makes anatomically accurate models and illustrations of the genitals with a focus on genital diversity—I wish we'd had these educational materials in school!

THE VULVA

I sat down with a hand mirror and properly looked at my own vulva for the first time at age twenty-five. Twenty-five!

Even though for the longest time I too referred to my entire external genitalia as the vagina, in fact, the correct name for it is the *vulva*. The vagina is actually only the internal canal—just that one specific part of the vulva—not the whole thing.

I had lived a quarter of a century without ever having actually taken a close look at this beautiful and important part of my own body. Some people live their whole lives never having done this.

I've received messages from women and vulva-owners not just in their teens or twenties, but even in their thirties and forties, surprised to learn from my videos that we don't pee from the same opening that we menstruate from.

You've probably learned something in school about the internal reproductive organs, and how babies are made, but there's very little attention paid to the external genitals, particularly the vulva.

Because, after all, we're still very much given the message that for people with vulvas, sex should be about having babies, not orgasms.

But for people of all genders, the genitals are a gold mine of pleasure-potential. They're crackling with nerve endings, and virtually each part can have a unique role to play in the experience of sexual pleasure.

And let's not forget—pleasure is a primary motivation when it comes to why people have sex. Of the millions of people having sex at this very moment all around the world, a very small fraction is doing so with the express intention of having a child. In fact, far more people are probably concerned, instead, with how to ensure that the sex they're having for pleasure won't get them pregnant!

Also, this sex-is-primarily-for-reproduction view that vulva-owners, in particular, are fed so relentlessly by society, ignores and delegitimizes queer sexual experiences.

Sex between people with penises and sex between people with vulvas is just as legitimate as sex between a person with a penis and a person with a vulva.

When learning about the genitals, it's fundamental that we learn about pleasure, too, rather than just about reproduction. We'd then be much more receptive to information about safer-sex practices, and we'd have much more enjoyable sex lives.

So, on that note, let's take a look at the anatomy of the vulva, with a particular focus on pleasure.

The Vulva

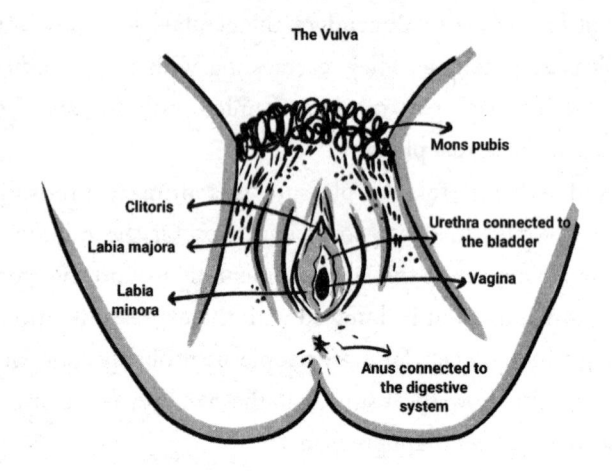

- Clitoris
- Labia majora
- Labia minora
- Mons pubis
- Urethra connected to the bladder
- Vagina
- Anus connected to the digestive system

Let's start from the top. The upside-down triangle of flesh below the stomach and between the tops of the thighs, where most of the pubic hair grows, is called the *mons*—the Latin word for mound or mountain.

The mons gives way to the *labia* or lips of the vulva—the outer lips are called the labia majora, and pubic hair grows here too. The inner lips comprise the thinner, darker, more crinkly folds of skin—the *labia minora*. The labia minora doesn't always appear symmetrical or 'tucked in'. And that's fine. For many people, it may have protruding or asymmetrical folds. Remember: *genital diversity is normal*, and your vulva is exquisite exactly the way it is.

The pea-shaped structure ensconced under a little hood of skin right where the mons first begins to part into the labia is the glans or head of the clitoris. It is central to the pleasure of

The Body

most vulva-owners, and regarded as the most reliable route to orgasm for many.

Below the external clitoris and above the vagina is a very small opening called the urethra. This is where we pee from. The urethra is also a sensitive region and thus may also contribute to pleasurable sensations for some people during sexual activity.

The larger opening below the urethra is the vaginal opening. The vagina is the internal canal that connects the vulva to the cervix and uterus. It is from the vagina that menstrual blood exits and from which a baby would exit during a vaginal delivery. It's where one would insert a tampon or a menstrual cup to collect period blood and where a penis would be inserted during penetrative vaginal intercourse.

Vaginal penetration with a penis, finger or sex toy may provide pleasure to some people with vulvas. However, most vulva-owners do not orgasm from penetration alone. External clitoral stimulation is also required. (More on the glorious clitoris in just a minute!)

Q How do I clean my vulva?

When it comes to keeping the vulva clean and healthy, it's important to remember that the vagina—the internal canal—is **a self-cleaning organ**, so you do not need to use soaps and cleansers inside it at all. In fact, even just excessive water going *inside* the vagina can upset its internal ecosystem and cause infections like Bacterial Vaginosis (BV).

And you don't actually need a special 'intimate wash'. You simply need to clean the external areas of the vulva—the mons, pubic hair, labia—with mild soap and water. Don't ever use any type of soap, cleanser or perfume *inside* your vaginal canal. You can use whatever body soap or shower gel you normally use for washing the external parts; it really doesn't require a special product.

When it comes to underwear, cotton is your best bet, as it's much more breathable than synthetic fabrics which can trap moisture and bacteria, especially when it's humid, or when you're exercising. For the same reason, wearing fresh undies each day, and changing out of wet swimsuits and sweaty gym clothes as soon as you're done is always a good idea.

Many of us worry about how we smell and taste 'down there', but it's important to understand that the vagina is not supposed to smell like strawberries or roses. It has its own natural scent and taste, and that's okay. If there's a sudden change in odour, or unusual discharge, then it might be worth seeing a doctor, but otherwise, the vagina's natural everyday scent and discharge are nothing to worry about. Most of us really need to learn to chill out about this during sex—instead of worrying about how we smell and taste, let's try to focus more on whether we're having a good time.

Here are some helpful tips I wish I hadn't learned the hard way:

Always pee after sex—it helps flush out bacteria that can otherwise easily enter the urethra and cause a urinary tract infection (UTI).

You don't want to put anything sugary on your vulva or vagina—save the Nutella for other parts of your body, if that's your thing. Anything sugary inside the vagina is a recipe for a yeast infection, which is a type of very common fungal infection. (Yeast infections can also occur as a side effect of taking antibiotics.)

Yeast infections, BV and UTIs are among the most common vaginal infections people experience—so common, in fact, that if you have a vagina, you are likely to experience each of them at some point in your life. Though they can be aggravated by sexual intercourse, they are not considered 'sexually transmitted infections' (STIs). People who aren't sexually active can also get them. And while they are no fun at all, luckily, they are totally treatable, and recovery is pretty swift.

Pay attention to things like soreness, itchiness, inflammation, redness, unusually thick discharge, or a burning sensation while peeing—these are often indications of an infection. The sooner you seek treatment, the sooner you'll be relieved of these rather uncomfortable symptoms. Don't delay the doctor's visit out of fear or embarrassment. It really isn't a big deal, and you don't want to wait till it gets unbearable. (Been there, done that, do not recommend!)

Q Should I get rid of my pubes?

Thanks to beauty standards set by pop culture and porn, as well as unexamined religious and cultural attitudes to personal hygiene, many people mistakenly believe that a hairless vulva is somehow 'cleaner' or 'better' than a hairy one—that it is 'healthy' to totally remove your pubic hair. This isn't true. It's simply an aesthetic choice, and it is worth noting the potential drawbacks.

Pubic hair exists for a reason—it cushions the genitals against friction and also serves as an initial barrier against bacteria and other unwanted pathogens.

In addition to eliminating these natural benefits, waxing can be incredibly painful, and shaving can lead to cuts. And both waxing and shaving can lead to itchiness, redness, soreness and infected hair follicles. Hair removal creams contain chemicals, and these too can cause irritation.

It is worth keeping these factors in mind instead of feeling pressurized to totally remove your pubic hair.

If you do want to get rid of it, remember, it is purely a matter of personal preference with regard to your own appearance. It is not something you owe anyone.

Personally, the approach I would recommend when it comes to pubic hair maintenance for people of any gender is trimming. Super-long pubes can do some annoying things sometimes, like get caught in the zippers of your pants on days you don't feel like wearing underwear, trap sweat after a workout, or take longer than you'd like to dry up after a shower. Simply trimming carefully with a small, clean pair of scissors, in my opinion, is the best of both worlds—you can keep things tidy without risking pain, rashes or infection.

Q Why is the skin around the genitals darker than the rest of my body?

For people of all genders, hormone changes during puberty cause the skin around the genitals and nipples to darken. It's also common for skin to be darker around the butt and inner thighs because these areas experience considerable friction during movement.

Hormonal changes during pregnancy as well as during the natural process of ageing may sometimes also impact the appearance or intensity of the colour of the skin on the genitals.

It's also normal for the colour of the genitals to intensify a little during sexual activity as a result of all the blood rushing to the area when you're sexually aroused—kind of like how your face might get a little red when you're flushed or blushing.

People often ask me if they should bleach their genitals. And my advice is, PLEASE DON'T. It can cause severe irritation and it isn't necessary.

Skin 'whitening' or 'fairness' products perpetuate the damaging, racist and colonial idea that fair skin is better or superior. I wish brands would stop making and marketing these products. They target people of colour and are sold primarily in countries that are former colonies. It's infuriating and I hope we stop buying them.

The Clitoris

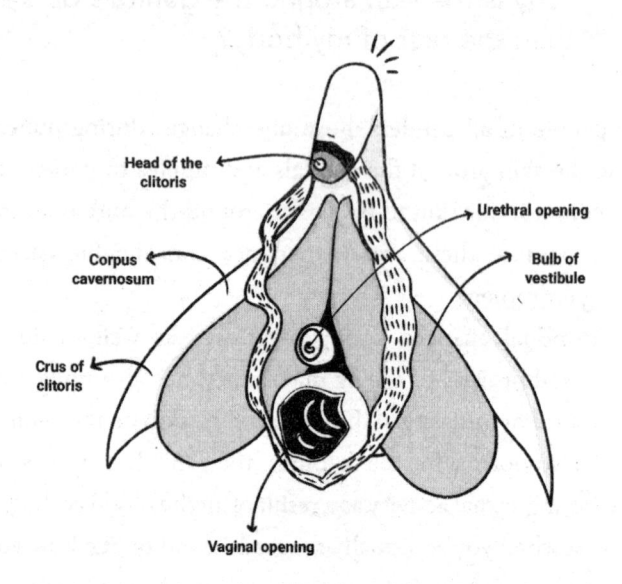

Head of the clitoris

Urethral opening

Corpus cavernosum

Bulb of vestibule

Crus of clitoris

Vaginal opening

The little nub at the top of the vulva that most people think of as the clitoris is actually only the *glans* or head of the clitoris. It is the area with the most nerve endings, and it's extremely sensitive to touch. It is a literal treasure trove of joyful possibilities. So central, in fact, is the clitoris to our pleasure that most people with vulvas don't experience orgasm from penetration alone. Clitoral stimulation is also required.

Just as focused, consistent stimulation of the penis is the most reliable route to orgasm for people with penises, focused, consistent stimulation of the clitoris is a one-way ticket to orgasm for most vulva-owners.

If you recall from earlier on in the book—the penis and the clitoris are homologous structures—they originate from the exact same tissue and share many similarities, including that they both play essential roles in the experience of sexual pleasure.

Yet, while stimulation of the penis is what we've been taught to basically centre heterosexual sex on, clitoral stimulation is thought of as optional—if it is thought of at all.

Also, the glans, or what we think of as the clitoris, isn't even the whole clitoris; it's just the tip of the iceberg, as it were. The bulk of the clitoral body actually extends internally such that its paired crura and vestibular bulbs straddle the vaginal canal. This is why external clitoral stimulation and internal vaginal stimulation—both at the same time—can feel ahhhhhmazing (more on this in a second).

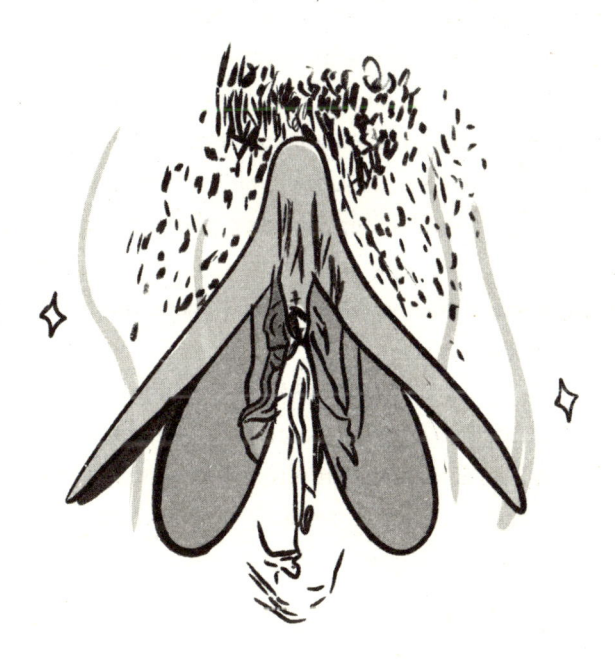

Unfortunately, the sexual anatomy and pleasure of vulva-owners haven't been a major priority in science labs for very long. It was only around 1998 that the structure of the internal clitoris became widespread, thanks to the work of Australian scientist Helen O'Connell, who published subsequent findings in 2005.

As humans, we've had the same anatomy for millennia but, especially when it comes to the science behind the pleasure of women and vulva-owners, we've only recently started to consider it worthy of far-reaching public discussion.

Q How do I find the G-spot?

I get this question a lot. *What* and *where* is the mystical G-spot? Named after German physician Ernst Gräfenberg, the G-spot has for decades been characterized by women's magazines and sex-advice books as if it's an elusive magic bean or button located somewhere on the upper wall of the vagina, leaving people very perplexed about what it is, where it is, and how to find it.

Well, it turns out there's no special magic bump or gland inside the vaginal canal.

In 2020, *Cosmopolitan* magazine even published a massive apology for perpetuating, for decades, the misconception that the G-spot is an actual separate physical structure to look for.

More recent scientific research shows that what was thought of as the 'G-spot' is, in fact, not a specific separate organ or gland at all—the walls of the vaginal canal are simply a sensitive *region*. The G-spot is **an erogenous zone**, not a distinct physical structure.

The arms that make up the internal structure of the clitoris straddle the urethra and the vaginal canal. So stimulation of the vagina, and especially the upper or anterior wall of the vagina (the vaginal wall closest to your belly), can feel particularly pleasurable because of the proximity of this part of the vaginal canal to the internal parts of the clitoris as well as the urethra right above it.

The clitoris and the urethra ensconce the vaginal walls: All these sensitive parts are located so close together—it makes sense that prodding and rubbing up against them can feel really intense!

The resulting sensitive area is 'the G-spot'. But it might have been more accurate to call it the G zone or G-region because 'spot' has too often been mistakenly construed as a separate, specific structure to look for.

More contemporary researchers have thus renamed the 'G-spot' the 'clito-urethro-vaginal complex'.[2] It's a mouthful to say, but it makes much more sense in that it accurately describes what's actually going on.

---

2   'Beyond the G-spot: Clitourethrovaginal Complex Anatomy in Female Orgasm', Emmanuele A. Jannini, Odile Buisson, Alberto Rubio-Casillas,
    https://pubmed.ncbi.nlm.nih.gov/25112854/

The Clito-Urethro-Vaginal (CUV) Complex

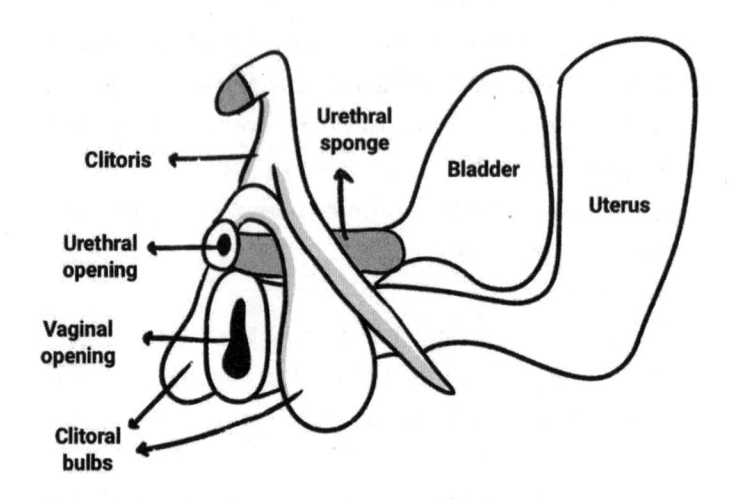

Diagram labels: Clitoris, Urethral opening, Vaginal opening, Clitoral bulbs, Urethral sponge, Bladder, Uterus

While most people with vulvas do require some amount of external clitoral stimulation to orgasm, and find clitoral stimulation very pleasurable even on its own, many find a combination of simultaneous external clitoral and internal vaginal stimulation exceedingly pleasurable—which makes sense when you understand the 'G-spot' as the clito-urethro-vaginal complex: stimulating the upper vaginal wall can indirectly stimulate the internal parts of the clitoris as well!

For example, many of us enjoy receiving oral sex on the external clitoris and fingering inside the vagina at the same time—and similarly, vibrators that provide both external clitoral and internal 'G-spot' stimulation simultaneously are especially popular.

That said, some people also like just vaginal penetration—the whole vaginal region and especially the upper wall *is* very sensitive for many vulva-owners and, for some, stimulation of that region *can* feel very pleasurable on its own too.

Often when a vulva-owner is close to orgasm, it can feel like you need to pee—and now this makes more sense too, right? Look at how close the urethra is to all the action!

People with vulvas experience pleasure in a huge variety of ways. But for too long we've been fed inaccurate information about our bodies—so it's no wonder our pleasure can seem puzzling. Hopefully, things are starting to make more sense for you as you read this book.

I have several videos on my Instagram and YouTube that showcase this anatomy using a life-size educational model of the vulva—go check them out! Now would be a great time, as they're likely to really drive home what you've just read, visually!

The Hymen Myth

Another misconception that has shrouded our understanding of our genital anatomy is the hymen myth. Most people think the hymen is a wall covering the vagina that 'breaks when a woman has sex for the first time', and that if a woman is a 'virgin', she 'ought to bleed the first time she has sex' because of it—that the hymen is somehow 'proof' of 'a woman's virginity'. This is simply not true.

'Virginity' itself is a ridiculous construct, and the idea that it can be 'proved' anatomically is unscientific garbage. The prevalent view of how the hymen works and the heavily gendered associations with 'virginity', 'purity', and 'honour' are a misunderstanding that has had dire, even fatal, consequences.

Contrary to what most people think, the hymen is a stretchy tissue, much less like a wall and much more like a scrunchie, that usually only partially covers the vaginal opening.

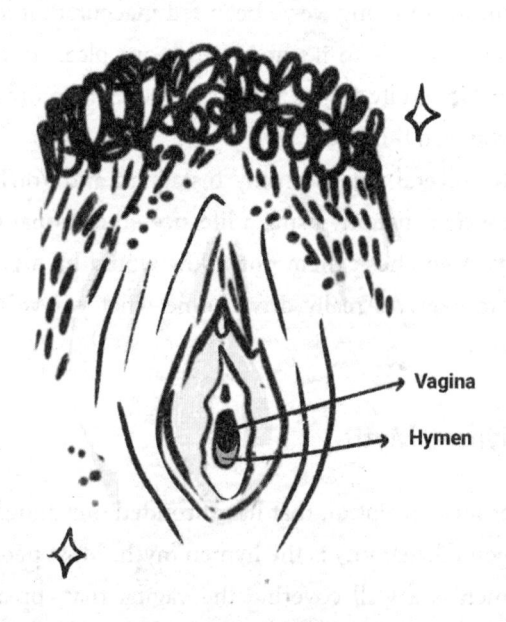

Even though we know that menstrual blood exits the vagina, and that a finger can easily be inserted, many people still mistakenly believe that the hymen is some sort of barrier that totally seals the vaginal opening, and that it breaks dramatically the first time one has penetrative sex. (Hence even the problematic 'insertion taboo' in many parts of the world, including our own, that persists around the use of products like tampons and menstrual cups.)

The truth is that the hymen is an elastic tissue, and while many of us have a sort of crescent-shaped hymen like in the diagram above, the amount of hymenal tissue present can vary. Some people are even born without a hymen, while others may have considerable hymenal tissue long after they begin being sexually active.

An imperforate hymen—where the hymen totally covers the vaginal opening—is a rare condition that requires surgery: because even menstrual blood cannot exit the body in such a case.

Hymens can vary

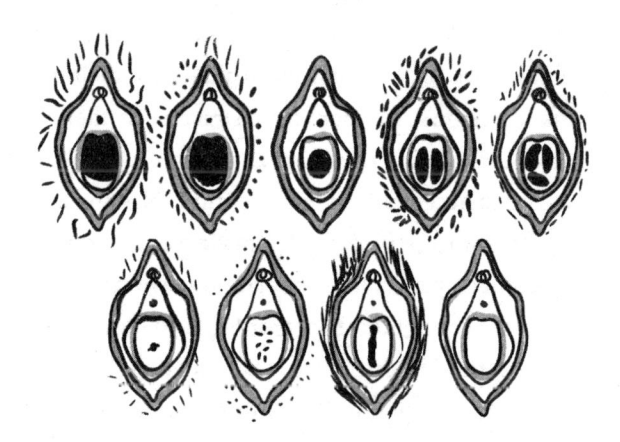

Because the amount of hymenal tissue varies from person to person, some people bleed when they first have penetrative vaginal intercourse, while others don't. I didn't.

When there is bleeding, it is often the result of insufficient lubrication and excessive friction which can cause vaginal tearing, rather than the stretching or rupturing of hymenal tissue alone.

Yet, for centuries, because of the dangerous, sexist mythology that surrounds the anatomy of the hymen, and a preoccupation with controlling and policing women's bodies and sexual autonomy, women have not only been slut-shamed and ostracized, but even killed for 'not bleeding on their wedding night'.

'Virginity tests' are also a patriarchal fabrication, and doctors or hospitals that claim they can provide such a test are frauds. There is no way to conclusively determine whether someone is a virgin by checking the hymen.

Whether a person has had sex or not, how many partners they may have had, whether or not a vulva-owner bleeds the first time they have sex—is no one's business but their own.

To link a person's 'honour' or 'character' to their sexual behaviour or the status of their hymen is not just misogynistic, regressive and unacceptable, it's unscientific, false and absurd.

We've also got to rethink the language we use around first sexual experiences, particularly in relation to women.

Consider the connotations of words like 'deflower' or 'pop her cherry', or the Hindi phrase *'seal todna'* (seal breakage) or even the very phrasing of *'losing* one's virginity'. In reality, nothing is 'lost', and while our first time having sex may be significant for many of us, there isn't some sort of dramatic 'biological' change to our bodies; it doesn't make you 'damaged goods'. A much more pleasant phrase, for example, that's become popular on social media, is 'sexual debut'. I'm glad we're looking for, and finding, more respectful and positive ways in which to talk about first-time sex!

Q Does sex make the vagina loose?

Kind of like the hymen myth, another myth used to slut-shame women is that of the 'loose vagina': The idea that if a woman has a lot of sex, she becomes a 'loose' woman, with 'loose' morals and a 'loose' vagina.

But that's another bunch of absolute nonsense. Sex does not make the vagina loose.

Somehow, people think that if a woman has sex with a hundred men, her vagina will become loose, but if she has sex with her husband a hundred times this won't happen. This itself proves the fallacy.

So here are some much better questions to consider:

How come when my girlfriend is really aroused, penetration can occur pretty easily, but if she's stressed or distracted about something else when we're trying to have sex, it's difficult to get my penis in? It feels like her vagina opens up when she's really excited, and is clamped shut when she's anxious or thinking of other stuff. Is this normal? – *Rishabh*

How come the vagina can have something as big as a baby come out of it and yet also be capable of holding something as tiny as a tampon in place all day? How come tampons or menstrual cups don't just fall out? – *Shai*

The vagina is an amazing organ which can change in response to hormones, life stages and physical and mental stimuli.

Indeed, the vaginal muscles relax when aroused. When a person with a vagina is turned on, the vaginal tissue typically becomes engorged with blood and produces additional lubrication. These are temporary states that the body assumes in response to sexual arousal.

On the flip side, if a person experiences fear or anxiety, the vaginal muscles will tighten temporarily. In either case, these are simply the body's natural (temporary) responses.

The muscles resume their original state when the feeling of arousal or the feeling of anxiety dissipates.

Let's now get to the second question. What makes the vagina so incredibly elastic is that its walls are covered by many folds called *rugae*. When the vagina is in its default state, its stretchy walls are flattened against each other by the pressure of the surrounding pelvic organs. The vagina therefore offers moveable support and pressure—it can easily stretch to accommodate something small like a tampon or menstrual cup when inserted, while also securely holding it in place.

The Vaginal Canal

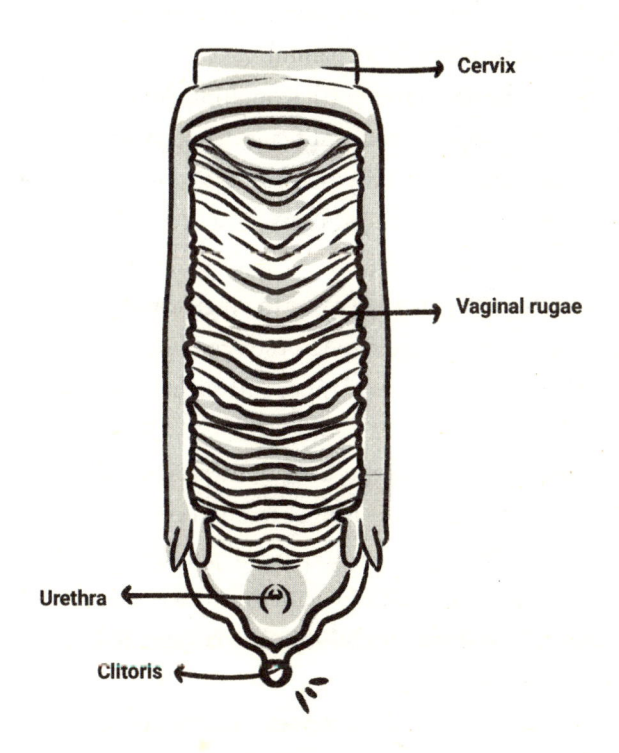

- Cervix
- Vaginal rugae
- Urethra
- Clitoris

As for how something as big as a baby can exit the vagina, the rugae enable the vagina to stretch and expand—kind of like how an accordion or a paper fan can unfold—when pressure is exerted against the vaginal walls, such as when a baby is being delivered vaginally.

Also, during pregnancy, the vagina responds to important changes in hormone levels. Throughout a pregnancy, the connective tissue of the vaginal walls progressively relaxes in preparation for childbirth. And despite all these incredible mechanisms of the vaginal anatomy, childbirth via vaginal delivery can be notoriously painful.

People who have given birth to multiple children via vaginal delivery, or who have had a difficult delivery, may experience decreased vaginal elasticity due to muscle fatigue or muscle tearing. However, in most cases, just a few months after delivery, the region heals.

The other thing that can cause the vaginal muscles to loosen slightly over time is ageing. As oestrogen levels may diminish with age, the vaginal walls may become slightly thinner and less elastic.

So let's get this straight: Sexual intercourse, masturbation with a toy or fingers, or using a tampon or a menstrual cup cannot cause the vagina to 'stretch out' permanently.

The only things that can actually impact vaginal elasticity are **multiple or difficult childbirths via vaginal delivery** and **the natural process of ageing**.

In either case, **Kegel exercises** can help, especially if you experience difficulty controlling bladder movements and other related issues.

Kegel exercises are simple exercises to **strengthen the pelvic floor muscles** which are the group of muscles that support the bladder, the uterus, the vagina and the bowels. You can look them up if you'd like to learn how to do them.

And while there's nothing wrong with strengthening your pelvic floor, it's also worth considering that the 'loose vagina' stigma has far more to do with how society likes to shame women for being sexual, as well as fetishize female youth, rather than any medically legitimized vaginal hierarchy.

Vulvas and Orgasms

I'm a 38-year-old woman, married with two kids. I've been having sex with my husband for over 10 years, but I don't think I've ever had an orgasm. – *Mariyam*

I'm pretty sure I've never had an orgasm. Sex with my boyfriend can be fun and I don't mind it, but I don't think I've ever experienced that ecstatic, moaning, out-of-control-climax-state or whatever it's called—that some of my friends tell me they've experienced and that women seem to experience all the time in porn and movies. – *Nikita*

Why do women take so much longer than men to orgasm? I want to ensure my girlfriend is enjoying herself when we have sex, but penetration seems to be more like a chore for her as opposed to something that makes her feel good. And it takes forever to make her come. Even then, I often wonder, maybe she's faking it just to get it over with. Help! I want our sex life to be as fun for her as it is for me. – *Rahul*

Across studies, globally, when people are asked whether they orgasm during sex with their partner, most straight men, most gay men, and most lesbians, report that they usually or always orgasm during sex. Straight women are the least likely to be able to say the same.

The Orgasm Gap

Research shows that within heterosexual couples, women tend to have significantly fewer orgasms than men. This disparity of orgasms is called the **orgasm gap**. If you're a straight woman, you probably don't need any convincing of this fact—you'll have most likely experienced this disparity yourself.

It's worth considering that most women report being able to orgasm during masturbation, as well as that women in relationships with women report significantly more frequent orgasms than women in relationships with men.

Are women's orgasms really so impossibly hard to figure out or are straight couples just not making women's pleasure a big enough priority? How do we bridge the gap?

Dr Laurie Mintz, author of the wonderful book *Becoming Cliterate: Why Orgasm Equality Matters—And How To Get It*, has some revealing statistics on how staggering the orgasm gap can be in experiences of heterosexual intimacy: 'When masturbating, 95% of women orgasm. In first-time hook-ups with other women, they orgasm 64% of the time. In first-time hook-ups with men, they orgasm 7% of the time. This tells us that the problem isn't women's ability to orgasm. It's our cultural scripts for heterosexual sex.'

Imagine if we got into elevators without knowing we had to press the buttons, or if we got into cars without knowing we needed the keys. That is literally how most straight men approach sex in relation to women's pleasure—without knowing enough about the clitoris.

And while Dr Laurie's research notes that the orgasm gap in heterosexual partnerships is maximum in first-time hook-ups, it reduces in friends-with-benefits equations, and shrinks further still in long-term relationships—presumably because the man becomes better acquainted with the woman's pleasure over time—it never closes. Not by a long shot.

This is in large part due to the fact that heterosexual sex tends to be seen as a penis-centric activity: erection, penetration, ejaculation. And the sex typically ends when he comes. Her orgasm seems optional at best.

When women have sex with other women, it's penetration that's optional. And when women masturbate, most choose to stimulate their external clitoris, either solely or coupled with penetration.

While the clitoris has been neglected for too long, and I think it is really important that we all learn about it, do remember that the specificities of each individual's pleasure preferences are unique—and one of the great joys of a shared sexual experience is discovering and celebrating those intricacies.

Some people may prefer indirect stimulation of the clitoris, such as touching it over their underwear or with a thin sheet or towel in-between. And there are also some vulva-owners who may not enjoy clitoral play quite as much and instead prefer penetrative stimulation or breast play or any number of other forms of stimulation.

Ultimately, communicating with your partner about their as well as your pleasure is the most important step to more satisfying, pleasurable sex.

Anorgasmia

A small percentage of people experience anorgasmia—an inability to orgasm despite sufficient stimulation. This is more common among women than among men. Physical factors such as childbirth, infection, surgery, chronic illness or pelvic floor muscle issues, as well as psychological factors like trauma or shame, can contribute to anorgasmia. It's worth seeing a doctor if this sounds like something you're going through.

Resist feelings of inadequacy or frustration if you're unable to orgasm. Be kind to yourself as you navigate your body and pleasure. Sex need not be goal-oriented—there's more to sex than orgasm—and you may find sexual intimacy very enjoyable nonetheless.

Pain During Sex

Is sex painful for women, specially the first time? – *Tamara*

I thought sex was supposed to feel good; is it normal for it to hurt? – *Niyati*

What should I do if penetration is painful for me? – *Divya*

We are often dismissively told that sex just *is* painful for women, as if it's simply one more thing on the long list of inconveniences that we have no choice but to put up with as women. But unless you're enjoying some consensual BDSM, sex should not be painful for anyone. And going through with sex when it is painful should not be expected of people of any gender.

Often pain during penetrative sex is a result of too much friction or not enough arousal and lubrication.

It certainly helps to take your time building up your arousal and sense of relaxation before attempting penetration. Activities traditionally considered 'foreplay', like kissing, touching, snuggling, tickling, eye gazing, massages, oral sex, manual stimulation, and breast and nipple play, can help you and your partner feel more and more relaxed and aroused.

It is also a great idea to use a store-bought personal lubricant—also known colloquially as 'lube'. Lube isn't just for older people, or people who experience severe vaginal dryness. Lube is for everyone. It's slippery and slidey, and it can make sex (and even masturbation) more comfortable and more fun for everyone, regardless of gender.

Vaginismus and Vulvodynia

For some people with vulvas, however, even after a lot of foreplay, and despite using lube, penetrative sex can be impossibly painful. Recurrent or persistent pain during penetrative sex could be an indication of an underlying condition like vaginismus or vulvodynia, and it is worth looking into with a doctor, as treatments exist.

Vaginismus is characterised by involuntary spasms of the pelvic floor muscles, making penetrative sex or even inserting something like a tampon into the vagina difficult, painful, or even impossible.

Vulvodynia affects the vulvar tissue—the external genitals and the area surrounding the entrance to the vagina. Some women have hypersensitive pain receptors in their vulvas which can make any contact or touch to the genitals very painful.

The research is limited on sexual pain disorders faced by people with vulvas and, sadly, they often go undiagnosed or misdiagnosed. They can be caused by a range of both physical and psychological factors.

Medical treatments are typically focused on alleviating symptoms, such as through topical or oral medications to relieve pain. Physical therapy and the use of vaginal dilators can help relax the tissue in the pelvic floor. A partner can also wear modular rings on their penis to ensure only a comfortable length is insertable during penetration.

For people living with sexual pain disorders, thoughts like 'what if it hurts me even more if we try to have sex again', or 'what if my partner breaks up with me because of this', as well as how one's partner responds—for example, if they feel inadequate, or if they coax you to try to go through with penetration anyway—can add to the discomfort already associated with sex because of the condition.

So, in addition to exploring physical and medical treatments, it is also worth exploring therapy and couples counselling with a mental-health professional.

Living with these conditions doesn't mean you can't have an enjoyable intimate life. Treatments may vary in duration and efficacy, depending on each individual's circumstances, but in the meantime, engaging in non-penetrative sexual activities and/or outercourse can be surprisingly pleasurable.

UNDERSTANDING HOW PERIODS AND PREGNANCY WORK

Now that we know about the external genitals of vulva-owners, I think I owe you some information about the internal reproductive functions, even though the focus of this book is pleasure.

Because, while pleasure is a significant, if not primary, motivation for why people have sex, and the area I'm personally most interested in writing about, reproduction is another important incentive for many, as well as a potential consequence or risk of heterosexual sex that many of us have to navigate in our pursuit of pleasure.

So, if you or your partner has a uterus, whether you want to figure out how to avoid pregnancy, or you're eager to become parents, understanding this stuff is definitely worth your while.

Let's jump right in.

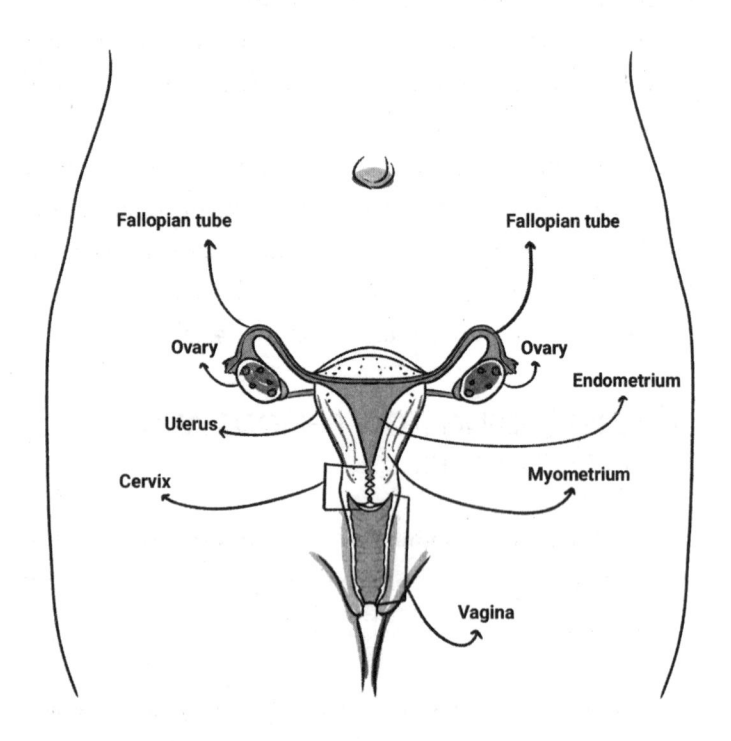

Fallopian tube — **Fallopian tube**
Ovary — **Ovary**
Endometrium
Uterus
Myometrium
Cervix
Vagina

Q What exactly has to happen for someone to get pregnant?

When people have sex to get pregnant, a person with a penis ejaculates inside a person with a vagina, both hoping that

The Body

conception—the fertilization of an egg by sperm—will take place.

We'll learn about sperm and testes when we get to the external genitals of penis-owners in just a bit. But for now, let's learn about where the eggs are, and how they are produced.

The ovaries are a pair of oval-shaped glands located on either side of the uterus that are responsible for the production of eggs and hormones. Ovulation occurs when an ovary releases an egg into an oviduct also known as the Fallopian tubes. Each ovary releases an egg alternately every month.

The oviducts or Fallopian tubes are the tunnels via which the egg cells travel from the ovaries to the uterus. Conception, or the onset of pregnancy—meaning the fertilization of an egg by sperm—usually occurs in these tubes.

While many of us might mistakenly think that a person with a uterus can get pregnant any day of the month, in fact, pregnancy is possible only around the time of ovulation. However, while eggs can be fertilized up to around twenty-four hours after they are released, sperm can live in a vulva-owner's reproductive tract for up to five days. Thus, many couples seeking to become parents often try to track ovulation by paying close attention to the vulva-owner's menstrual cycle, scheduling sex on the days leading up to ovulation.

Unfortunately, estimating your cycle absolutely perfectly and figuring out exactly which days you're most likely to be 'fertile' and which days you're not, is easier said than done. We're only 'fertile' for a few days every month, with our fertility declining as we get older. This means getting pregnant can often be quite a lot harder than it sounds when a couple actually starts having sex with the intention to get pregnant—but, ironically, it's also why accidental pregnancies are very common too. Preventing pregnancy without using protection is quite a lot harder than it sounds. If you're not trying to get pregnant, I'd recommend you always use protection.

But back to the eggs. If an egg is fertilized, it moves to the uterus, where it implants itself in the endometrium, or inner lining of the uterus, that has been prepped for its arrival. The uterus is the organ that is colloquially referred to as the 'womb'. When a pregnancy occurs, it serves as home to the developing foetus.

Q Okay, so what is a period?

If an egg is not fertilized by sperm, it disintegrates in the fallopian tube within a few days. The endometrial tissue is then shed along with blood, and secretions from the vagina and cervix, as a 'period'.

While most people think that the **menstrual cycle** is just the few days of monthly bleeding, or the 'period', in fact, the menstrual cycle is the entire span from the first day of your period till the first day of your next period, which is roughly a month.

And, as you may have figured out from what you've read here so far, it's actually made up of two cycles that interact and overlap—one occurring in the ovaries and the other taking place in the uterus.

The first part of the cycle gets an egg ready to be released from the ovary and prepares the lining of the uterus. The second part of the cycle lays the groundwork for the body to accept a fertilized egg, or to shed the endometrial tissue and start the next cycle if pregnancy doesn't occur.

A complex interaction of hormones serves as a sort of communication system between the brain, ovaries and uterus to keep the menstrual cycle going.

In the event that an egg is successfully fertilized and implanted, these hormones facilitate the complex choreography of maintaining and nurturing a pregnancy over roughly nine months, from conception to delivery.

If you don't get pregnant, the body sheds the uterine lining and basically preps itself to try again with a new egg every month until **menopause**. (Unlike sperm which keeps being produced in the testes, people with ovaries are born with a finite supply of eggs—so we eventually have none left, and we stop getting our period and being able to get pregnant. More on menopause in a moment.)

If you skipped a period, does it mean you're pregnant?
– *Ankita*

If you're pregnant, you don't get your period; hence a skipped period can be an overwhelming event. For many people, it's how they first discover they may be pregnant.

However, pregnancy isn't the only possible reason for a missed period. Stress, hormonal imbalance, weight change, strenuous exercise, the onset of menopause and other varied factors can lead to menstrual irregularities too. Many people have also reported menstrual irregularities after having had COVID-19, as well as soon after getting the vaccines.

If you have been sexually active and you've missed a period, it's certainly worth seeing a gynaecologist (gynac). You can take a pregnancy test at the gynac's clinic or even in the safety and privacy of your own bathroom.

If you test positive, your gynac can help you determine what your options are, and you can make the choice that's right for you. If you test negative, but you still don't get your period after a while, again, your gynac can help you determine the cause of and possible solutions to the menstrual irregularities you may be experiencing.

Period Sex: Yay or Nay?

I get really horny on my period, but I'm grossed out by the idea of period sex and my boyfriend is even more grossed out. Period blood just seems super disgusting! Is it okay to have sex when you have your period? – *Clarissa*

Many people are uncomfortable with the idea of period sex. Some spout archaic beliefs from religious texts to claim that it's 'bad' or 'wrong' and that it makes you 'impure' or 'immoral'. Others think it must be unhealthy, unhygienic or harmful.

Most of us are just so steeped in the social stigmas surrounding female sexuality and menstruation, and the shame we learn to feel around the body, that we haven't really thought it all through, and we're scared or disgusted by the idea of period sex by default.

It's an unexamined and often misogynistic disgust with a natural bodily function, rather than any really solid reasoning, that makes people squirm at the thought of period sex.

So let's break it down. It is perfectly fine to have period sex. Some menstruators experience a higher desire for sex during their period, and sexual pleasure can even relieve menstrual cramps and headaches. There is nothing immoral about having sex on your period—it may actually provide some relief!

That said, of course, there are many people who simply don't feel like having sex on their period, and that's absolutely fine too. When I'm on my period, I often just want to curl up with a hot water bottle and some snacks, and be cranky. There's no pressure to have sex.

It's just worth understanding that period sex isn't objectively wrong, 'gross', or harmful, and many people even find it to be rather enjoyable.

Let's take this opportunity to remind ourselves that menstruation is a normal and, in fact, absolutely vital part of human existence. And no matter our gender, it's worth overcoming any feelings of shame or disgust around it.

Q Is it safe to have unprotected sex on your period?

We're so confused about whether to have sex when I'm on my period or not—on the one hand, it's the one time in the month I can be sure I won't get pregnant if we do it without protection, right? On the other hand—can't you get infections from period blood? – *Ria*

First of all, you *could* get pregnant even when on your period. Sperm can live in the body for up to five days; and different people's ovulation cycles vary in duration—so, although unlikely, it is not impossible. (Also, some people may bleed even during ovulation, or may experience vaginal bleeding for a different reason and mistake it for a period.)

If you want to avoid pregnancy, and you are not on any other form of birth control, it's best to always use condoms, even when on your period.

As for infections—period blood isn't inherently diseased or dirty; if you don't have an infection, an infection won't be transmitted. However, period sex can increase the chance of transmission if an infection is present.

If you and your partner haven't both been tested for sexually transmitted infections, it's best to always use a barrier method of protection, whether or not you have your period, and whether or not you're also on some other form of birth control.

Remember that while contraceptives like birth control pills and IUDs (intrauterine devices) work to prevent pregnancy, only barrier methods like condoms and dental dams give protection against the transmission of infection.

Q If you have had unprotected sex, can you take a pregnancy test the same day?

Whether you are someone who wants to get pregnant or someone who is hoping you don't get pregnant, it's understandable that you'd want to know what's going on ASAP.

But home pregnancy tests aren't going to be able to tell you on the same day. It's too early for an accurate result. Most home pregnancy tests can be done from the first day of your missed period. If you're not sure when you're having your next period—or if your period is irregular—it's generally suggested that you take the test at least ten days after you had unprotected sex.

If you had unprotected sex and you don't want to become pregnant, you can take emergency contraception, also often referred to as the 'morning-after pill'.

With emergency contraception on the other hand, the sooner you are able to take it after having sex, the more likely it is to be able to work. Emergency contraception is best taken as soon as possible—ideally on the same day or by the next day—and it's not considered effective if taken later than five days after intercourse.

It's best to use a primary form of contraception such as condoms, birth control pills, or an IUD if you're sexually active and do not wish to get pregnant—emergency contraceptives are less effective at preventing pregnancy than a primary method of contraception, and therefore should ideally be thought of as a recourse for when a primary method failed or was not in place, rather than as your go-to for contraception. You'll find lots more on protection and contraception when we get to the chapter on safety (see page 124).

Premenstrual Syndrome (PMS) and Premenstrual Dysphoric Disorder (PMDD)

What exactly is PMS? Why do I feel so irritable and bloated and sensitive right before my period? – *Tamanna*

In the lead up to my period, even the silliest things like cheesy adverts, that would ordinarily be utterly unable to move me, can push me to tears, and people's otherwise innocuous quirks—chewing loudly, or asking unnecessary questions—can make me snap. I feel bloated, and yet I want cake, and I also want to bite everyone's head off. I sometimes even experience feelings of total hopelessness. I know I'm about to get my period when I am suddenly overwhelmed by the seeming pointlessness of life. And I know I'm not alone.

Every month when I feel this way, my mum reminds me with the same joke:

'Leez, why do they call it PMS?'

'Why, mom?'

'Because Mad Cow Disease was already taken.'

Most menstruators experience at least mild symptoms of PMS in the lead-up to their period, and sometimes even around the time of ovulation. Symptoms such as the ones I have just described, as well as some others.

Thanks to the cyclical hormonal changes taking place in our bodies to facilitate the menstrual cycle, we may experience mood changes, acne, sore breasts, irritability, emotional overwhelm, cramps, bloating, cravings, insomnia, fatigue—or all of the above.

If you menstruate, you probably know exactly what I'm talking about.

Premenstrual dysphoric disorder or PMDD is a more severe form of PMS, which fewer people experience, but which can be very debilitating. Changes in mood may feel more like depression and anxiety, and some people even experience suicidal thoughts.

Again, it's definitely worth talking to a gynaecologist if you experience such premenstrual symptoms, as there are lifestyle changes as well as medication that can make them far more manageable.

For too long, periods and PMS have been weaponized against menstruators, and period stigma remains one of the many symptoms of the misogyny that thrives in a patriarchal society. Instead, we deserve to be able to understand our bodies and have easy, affordable access to the healthcare and resources we may need.

In my late teens and early twenties, I was much less informed about the body—my school didn't have sex-ed either. I began tracking my period with a menstrual tracking app only in my mid-twenties—I wish I'd started sooner. I highly recommend using one if you menstruate—my personal favourite is an excellent app called Clue.

It can really help you make sense of what's going on in your body. Because even though things like those inexplicably angry pimples you get before your period, the headaches, bloating, tender breasts, mood swings, meltdowns or whatever other symptoms you experience—as well as your actual period—may seem random and therefore all the more annoying to you when you don't track your cycle, they're actually often surprisingly predictable once you begin paying closer attention.

Tracking my cycle has really helped me understand my own body and the hormonal roller coaster ride it goes through on a monthly basis. I'm now able to prepare for and manage my body's changing requirements, instead of having them catch me off guard.

Dysmenorrhea (Period Pain)

Many people experience painful periods, a condition called dysmenorrhea. Most often, period pain is caused by menstrual cramps, and feels like a throbbing pain in your lower abdomen. However, one may also have other symptoms, such as lower back pain, nausea and headaches.

So why are periods painful for some of us? There are two types of dysmenorrhea: primary and secondary, and each type has different causes.

Primary dysmenorrhea is the most common type of period pain. It is caused by the onset of menstruation itself and not by any other condition. Chemicals called prostaglandins (which work kind of like hormones) make the muscles of your uterus tighten and relax, and this causes the cramps. Some people may experience pain a day or two before their period.

Secondary dysmenorrhea is pain caused by something other than menstruation itself, most often by conditions that may affect the uterus or other reproductive organs, such as **endometriosis** and **uterine fibroids**. (Endometriosis is when tissue similar to the endometrium grows outside your uterus. Uterine fibroids are non-cancerous growths in the uterus.)

Pain isn't something you should have to grin and bear. Using a hot-water bottle or heat pad can feel very comforting, and many people find tremendous relief from simply taking an over-the-counter painkiller like ibuprofen, which doctors often recommend for period cramps. To manage conditions like endometriosis or uterine fibroids, a gynac can help you determine the most suitable course of action, be it medication, medical procedures, or monitoring and managing symptoms.

Polycystic Ovary Syndrome (PCOS)

I have very irregular periods, and am wondering if maybe I have PCOS/PCOD. What does 'polycystic' mean exactly and what is the difference between the two? Also, how do I know if I should see a doctor? – *Seher*

Polycystic ovarian syndrome (PCOS) and polycystic ovarian disease (PCOD) are a common cause of menstrual irregularities.

PCOS is the more contemporary parlance in an effort to move towards using language that isn't stigmatizing—such as the word 'disease'. Since PCOS comprises a collection of symptoms, 'syndrome' also encompasses that more effectively.

As the term 'polycystic' suggests, the condition is typically accompanied by the presence of fluid-filled sacs or 'cysts' in the ovaries. However, it's important to note that many people have cysts but don't have PCOS and, likewise, some people may not have cysts but still have PCOS.

With PCOS, the endocrine system is also impacted and therefore it is typically accompanied by symptoms such as significant hormonal imbalances, weight gain, acne, more facial and body hair, hair fall or baldness and, sometimes, infertility.

While there is no 'cure' for PCOS, fortunately, simple lifestyle changes such as modifications in diet and exercise can go a long way in managing symptoms.

As for medication: birth control pills may be prescribed to regularize periods, hormones for fertility, and hair growth inhibitors or hair-removal procedures may be prescribed to tackle increased facial or body hair.

So if you experience any such symptoms, it's worth consulting a gynac about PCOS, because the good news is there is a lot that can be done to manage and treat the symptoms. Plus, the earlier someone is diagnosed, the more effectively their condition can be managed.

While some people may have difficulty getting pregnant if they have PCOS, it's not impossible—so it's worth talking to your doctor about your options. Likewise, it's important to still use protection rather than see PCOS as an indication that you don't need to take precautions if you are not looking to get pregnant.

While the thought of being diagnosed with polycystic ovaries can sound scary, remember, it's nothing to be embarrassed or ashamed of. It is a common condition and can be effectively managed with relatively simple interventions.

DEBUNKING PERIOD MYTHS

'Periods make you impure'

In India, millions of menstruators drop out of school and miss out on opportunities in the workforce because of period stigma and a lack of access to menstrual hygiene resources. Many also face restrictions in participating in family life and in practising their faith during their period.

These taboos that stem from the idea that menstrual blood is somehow 'immoral' or 'impure' are unscientific, misogynistic and absurd. Pickles will not spoil, temples and kitchens will not be contaminated, you can wash your hair, you can play sport/exercise if you wish, you can eat whatever and wherever you choose, you can meet whomever you like, and you can have sex when you're on your period.

What you do or don't do while on your period should be a matter of personal choice, not a predetermined and oppressive social script. If you feel like taking a day off, that's fine; if you don't feel like exercising, that's fine. If you're not into temple visits in any case, that's fine. If you don't want to have period sex, no problem.

But we deserve to be able to make these choices based on how we feel on any given day, rather than have them made for us by the unscientific and misogynistic restrictions we're pressurized to adhere to simply because we're menstruating.

> ### 'Only Women Have Periods'
>
> Not all women menstruate. And not everyone who menstruates is a woman. Some cis women are born without a functional uterus and many have conditions due to which the uterus may need to be removed. And one cannot menstruate after menopause anyway. Trans women and trans feminine people do not have a uterus, while trans men and non-binary people with a uterus may experience menstruation. A period or the lack of it does not singularly define womanhood; gender identity is not contingent on whether or not you menstruate. This needs to be acknowledged.

Menstrual Hygiene Products

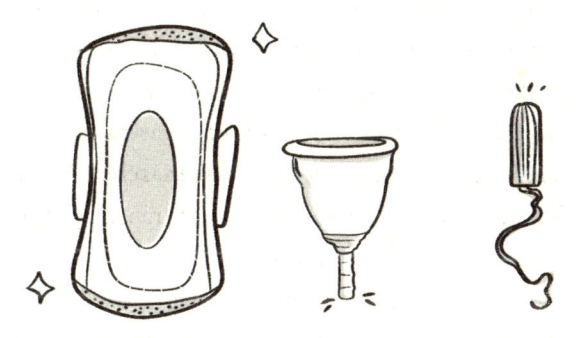

Using whatever menstrual products work for you is fine—there's no shame in using or not using a menstrual cup, for example. It's a great sustainable period product, and no, you can't 'lose your virginity' to a menstrual cup—but it also requires access to clean water to use, which not everyone has—and some people, for whatever reason, might prefer to use more traditional products like pads or tampons, which is fine too. You do you.

Menopause

I'm an unmarried woman who just turned 30 and now people are constantly telling me that my 'biological clock' is ticking. WTF does that mean? Maybe I do eventually want to have kids. But I'm not ready yet. How much time do I have? – *Riddhima*

People with ovaries are born with all the eggs their body will ever produce. Unlike with sperm, new eggs are not made during our lifetime. As we get older, the quality and supply of our eggs decline. We eventually run out of eggs and hence stop getting our periods. This natural cessation of menstruation is called menopause. Kind of like puberty and **menarche** (the onset of periods), menopause, too, is a process of transition. It usually occurs sometime between the ages of forty-five and fifty-five, but can occur before or after this age range too.

Menopause is often accompanied by symptoms like irregular bleeding, hot flashes and weight gain. These symptoms may begin a few years before one's last period and may continue for a few years after.

The stage of hormonal changes that signal the lead-up to menopause is called **perimenopause**, during which periods typically become irregular.

Menopause is usually marked by a full year without periods, and **post-menopause** refers to the years after menopause has occurred.

Menopause remains yet another normal bodily function that our society looks upon unfavourably. As an unmarried, childfree woman in my thirties myself, I get told my 'biological clock is ticking' all the time too.

Personally, I simply have no interest in having children, and I take offence at the suggestion that my primary purpose in life is unfulfilled if I don't become a mother, if I don't 'reproduce'.

I also believe we've got to reject the stereotypes around 'menopausal women' as 'over the hill', as somehow less 'feminine', bereft of 'desirability'. So to hell with my biological clock, as far as I'm concerned.

Still, I do realize that many people do want to have children—and if you do, it's helpful to understand the menstrual cycle, to acknowledge the inevitability of menopause and to take the decisions you need to in order to fulfil your own aspirations on your own timeline. Have a baby? Freeze your eggs? Adopt? Remain childfree? You get to decide what's right for you.

BOOBS

Q Does size matter?

All through my teenage years and well into my twenties, I was really self-conscious about my boobs. I thought they were too small; I would wear heavily padded bras; I even apologized to my partners in my first few relationships: mid make-out, as our shirts came off, I would hurry to say: 'I'm sorry my boobs are so small!' I would actually *apologize*—how sad and unnecessary is that? I wish I could go back in time and give myself a hug. The truth is: my boobs are delightful. And so are yours.

Unfortunately, we are conditioned from such a young age to think that a Barbie doll figure is the ultimate standard, that we should have big boobs, no tummy, a bubble butt and also a thigh gap. We internalize these totally unrealistic beauty standards and then have terrible self-esteem, constantly dissatisfied with our bodies and feeling as if we're not good enough.

Many women with small boobs wish they had bigger boobs because they think it would make them more attractive, but some women with big boobs also wish they had smaller boobs—big boobs can hurt your back and it can also be exhausting dealing with the unwanted attention they receive. (We have really got to stop staring at and commenting on people's boobs!)

All boobs are great boobs, whatever their size. Not only are they an absolutely beautiful form, capable of providing you with a lot of pleasure, they also have the capacity to nourish life—how magical! Even though I myself don't plan on having any children, I do think that's pretty amazing.

So, love your boobs. Look at yourself in the mirror and appreciate how lovely they are.

Accepting your body is a major step towards better self-esteem and happier relationships.

Q Why is one boob bigger than the other?

It's very likely that each of your breasts is a little bit different from the other.

Maybe one is a little bigger or rounder or pointier; maybe one boob is placed slightly higher or lower on your chest than the other. Maybe you've wondered whether you should freak out about it.

While stuff like pop culture, porn and magazine covers have misled many of us into believing that boobs should be perfectly round and symmetrical, guess what, *most* boobs are not.

For some people, the differences are subtle, while for others they might be more apparent. Many folks even have a whole cup size difference between their boobs. And that's fine!

Boobs, like most of the body parts that come in pairs are sisters, not twins.

If you look carefully at your hands, feet, eyes, ears, butt cheeks, or even, say, just the left side of your nose versus the right side, you'll notice that, in fact, perfect symmetry is present almost nowhere.

You probably have some fingers that are a bit less straight than others, one eye that's a bit bigger or droopier than the other, etc., etc., etc.

And it's these little asymmetries that make you look uniquely yourself.

It's no different for boobs. So embrace the asymmetries instead of freaking out about them.

A lot of what one's breasts look like is simply down to genetics—but fluctuations in weight can also impact boob size. When you gain or lose weight, it doesn't always happen perfectly uniformly all over your body. Also, stuff like breastfeeding can impact boob symmetry—all of this is nothing to be embarrassed or panic about.

Nipples and Areola

What do normal nipples look like? I feel mine are kind of big, and also there's sometimes a few hairs on them. Is this okay? – *Zainab*

Nipples come in a range of shapes and sizes. Some can be tiny and round, some are larger or more oblong, some are flatter or more protruding. Some people may have inverted nipples— nipples that turn inwards. It's all A-Okay!

The circular area of pigmented skin immediately around a nipple is called the **areola**.

Areolae can vary from the size of a coin to the size of a saucer, and the colour of nipples and areolae can vary from very light pink to very dark brown, and is often related to one's overall skin colour.

The size, shape and colour of nipples and areolae can also change gradually over the course of one's life, due to factors such as puberty, pregnancy, breastfeeding, menopause and general ageing.

As with boobs, there's a lot of variation and diversity when it comes to what nipples can look like and, again, that's normal!

Q Why do nipples get hard?

The nerves in the nipples react to stimuli, both physical and psychological. While sometimes it can be a response to arousal such as a sexual touch or thought, nipples getting hard isn't always or inherently sexual. It can also happen due to something as simple as change in temperature, such as when you feel cold, or even something as simple as the fabric of your shirt or undergarments brushing against your skin. So it's really no big deal and nothing to worry about — it's just the body being the body and doing its thing. And whether hard or not, so what if nipples are sometimes visible through your clothing—they're just a part of the body! It's something we shouldn't have to feel so conscious about.

Why It's Important to Examine Your Boobs

If you haven't really given much thought to the well-being of your boobs before, it's worth taking the time to familiarize yourself with how they normally look and feel.

Don't be alarmed—normal boob tissue does not feel like a perfectly smooth jelly, to begin with.

Here's what a boob's anatomy looks like inside:

The Anatomy of the Female Breast

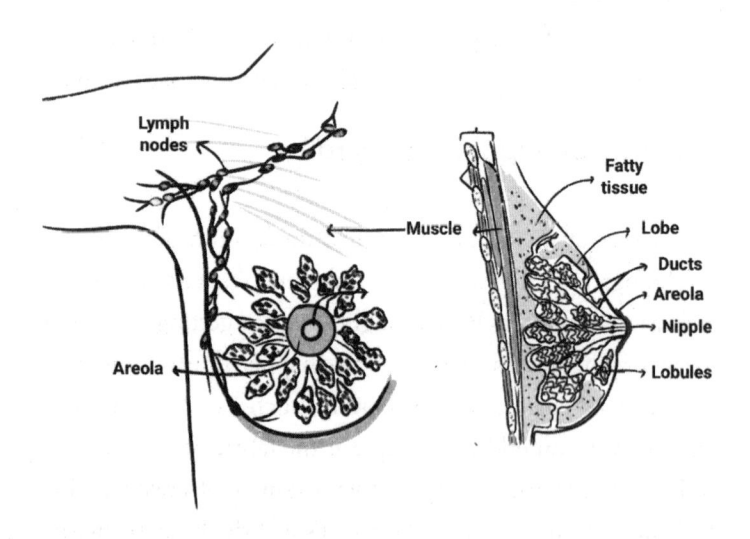

There are lots of milk glands and ducts under the skin that give it a unique texture. Hormonal variations and your menstrual cycle can also make your boobs feel bigger, or lumpier, and also sometimes cause soreness or tenderness.

Once you figure out what normal looks and feels like for you, make it a point to examine your boobs yourself once a month so that you notice in case something suddenly changes.

All you've got to do is stand in front of a mirror with your arms up, one at a time, using the pads of two fingers to check each breast and armpit area.

Look out for unusually lumpy or dimpled skin, changes in your skin colour or texture, and nipple deformation or discharge.

If you feel an unfamiliar lump or a sudden increase or decrease in the volume of a breast, especially if accompanied by other symptoms like skin retraction, thickening, dimpling, or a change in the colour of the skin on your breast, it's worth consulting a doctor, as changes like these can sometimes indicate breast cancer.

There's a very good possibility that it's nothing at all or that if there is anything, it's benign—but it's better to be safe than sorry.

Breast cancer is one of the most common forms of cancer—but it's also one of the most treatable, if detected early.

Let's learn to appreciate our boobs, whether big or small or asymmetrical and let's make sure we look after them!

THE PENIS

The external genitalia of people with penises comprises, you guessed it—the penis—with its glans or mushroom-shaped head, its shaft—the body or length of the penis—as well as the scrotum or ball sac which encases the testicles.

70   **THE SEX BOOK**

- Penis
- Testes (in scrotum)
- Glans
- Opening of urethra

Circumcised (Foreskin removed)

Uncircumcised (Foreskin present)

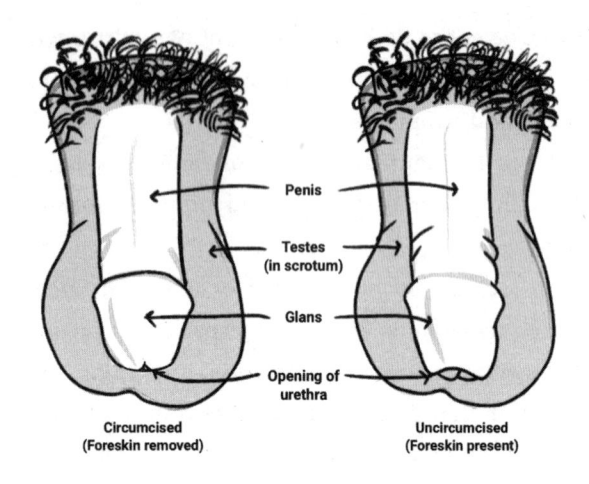

Penis Anatomy

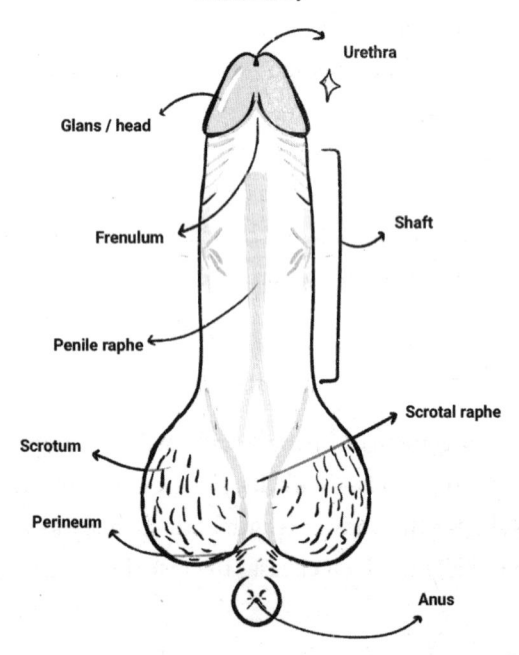

- Urethra
- Glans / head
- Frenulum
- Shaft
- Penile raphe
- Scrotal raphe
- Scrotum
- Perineum
- Anus

The glans is the head or tip of the penis. The opening of the urethra is located here, which is where urine, pre-cum and semen exit from. For many people, the glans is the most sensitive part of the penis. In an uncircumcised penis, the foreskin drapes over the head of the penis like a hood when not erect. When erect, the foreskin retracts and exposes the glans. In a circumcised penis, the foreskin is absent. This leaves the glans visible at all times, whether erect or not.

The shaft of the penis extends from the glans to where it connects to the lower belly or pubic region. The shaft houses the urethra and is made up of layers of spongy tissue which can fill up with blood when stimulated—this is what causes a penis to grow in size and firmness when erect.

A small ridge of skin called the frenulum connects the foreskin to the penis and the raphe is the line or seam along the underside of the shaft of the penis that extends across the scrotum and perineum as well.

At the start of the book, I explained how we all start off with the same genital tissue as foetuses. No matter whether you eventually have a penis or a vulva, everyone begins with a little genital tubercle, urogenital folds and a labioscrotal area that is fairly similar to 'female' genital anatomy. This then develops into a clitoris and labia, or transforms into a penis and scrotum upon exposure to the hormones produced during sexual differentiation. The penile and scrotal raphe is literally the seam where the folds fuse along the midline during sexual differentiation over the course of foetal development—a little reminder of our shared beginnings!

Penis Hygiene

What exactly is smegma, and how to keep the penis clean and healthy? – *Aman*

The penis and general pubic region can be washed daily with gentle soap and water. It's also best to wash up before and after sex, as well as after exercise, and to dry the area before wearing clothing.

Smegma is the white build-up that sometimes collects on the tip and under the foreskin of the penis, or in the folds of the vulva. Thus, an uncircumcised penis requires some extra attention to hygiene. If you don't regularly clean under the foreskin (gently, of course), bacteria, dead skin cells and oil can cause smegma.

By the way, keeping your penis 'healthy' also means using protection and getting checked for STIs, if you are sexually active.

Average Penis Size

What is the average penis size? How big does your penis need to be in order to satisfy your partner? – *Anurag*

Personally, I think there's no need to get fixated with numbers or averages, or seek to compare your own penis with anyone else's, but since so many people who write to me seem to want to know how long the 'average' penis is, here's what's generally said:

According to data from several studies on penis size, it appears that the average penis is around five inches in length when erect.[3]

Different people are built differently, even when it comes to their penises. There are 'growers' who tend to start small and end up bigger when erect and 'showers' who tend to start out big and not get much bigger when erect. As I keep saying, genital diversity is normal.

Q Does size matter?

Hundreds of men write to me every day with the same questions: **How can I make my penis bigger? How can I 'improve' my penis size? Is it possible to please your partner with a small penis?**

Here's my take: Don't worry so much about penis size. *Dil bada hona chaiye bas*. A big heart is all that matters.

Other than surgery, there's very little you can do to make the actual size of your penis bigger. Please don't fall for the numerous scams that prey on this body insecurity and try to

---

3 'Average-Size Erect Penis: Fiction, Fact, and the Need for Counseling', B.M. King, https://www.tandfonline.com/doi/full/10.1080/0092623X.2020.1787279

sell you lotions and potions with the promise of a bigger dick. No pills, creams, or oils can make your penis grow permanently.

As for Viagra—that's a medication that helps with erections. It doesn't increase your penis size and, like most medications, it has its own list of possible contraindications and side effects—it should only be used if a doctor has prescribed it.

I'm of the opinion that size really does not matter, and that we desperately need to rethink our views on sex and masculinity, which currently remain far too fixated on the penis and on **penetration**.

While penetration can feel good, as I've said repeatedly, it is worth remembering that the scripts we've been fed, particularly about heterosexual sex, are really very limiting and unimaginative and penis-centric. There is so much you can do to share and experience pleasure that has nothing at all to do with penetration and penis size.

Consider the fact that lesbians often report greater sexual satisfaction than women in relationships with men. This indicates that what matters far more than the size or even the presence of a penis is simply an understanding of your partner's body and arousal, and a willingness and enthusiasm to make their pleasure a priority.

Keep in mind, for example, that focused and consistent stimulation of the clitoris is the most reliable route to orgasm for most people with vulvas. Oral sex and fingering are among the most effective ways to provide clitoral stimulation, and have nothing to do with penis size. Plus, even for penetration, think about it—if a finger can work, you don't really need a super big penis for it to feel good. If you communicate with your partner, and ask them what they enjoy, you're probably going to be able to provide a LOT of pleasure no matter what size you are.

You can even enjoy mutual masturbation where you together touch yourselves exactly how you like to be touched—instead of always seeing sex as some sort of event where one partner must necessarily only do things to the other and vice versa.

It's also worth keeping in mind that the vagina and the anus are both relatively small orifices. So the idea that bigger is necessarily better when it comes to any type of penetrative sex is something of a misconception—a really big penis can even cause significant pain during sex.

Whatever your penis size, and whatever your sexual orientation, by simply communicating with your partner and giving equal priority to their pleasure, you can certainly find a lot of ways to please each other in bed.

And that brings me to my main point. Which is that a keen understanding of how bodies work in relation to pleasure, and qualities like enthusiasm and confidence and respect, have a far greater impact on the quality of a sexual experience than the size or appearance of any particular body part—for anyone of any gender or sexual orientation.

The fact is that the bodies we see in mainstream porn or movies or magazine covers or wherever else, are rarely representative of what most people's bodies look like.

Most people don't have massive penises, bulging biceps and ultra-defined abs, or big, perfectly round boobs, a tiny waist and a peach-like butt with no cellulite. Most people just aren't all shiny and sculpted and hairless and big in only the 'right' places.

And guess what? That's okay. Those arbitrary 'beauty standards' are best discarded. You don't have to look a certain way to experience pleasure. You simply need to approach sex with a sense of non-judgemental curiosity and playfulness and respect.

Curvature

My penis has a little bit of a curve to it when I'm hard. Is that normal? – *Savio*

It is very common for the penis to curve slightly to the right or left when erect. This is generally harmless and not a cause for concern.

However, a severe curve accompanied by pain during sex could indicate Peyronie's Disease (PD), which can sometimes make erections painful. PD develops when scar tissue forms inside the penis, usually due to an injury. If this sounds like a possibility, it's worth seeing a urologist to seek treatment.

Circumcised vs Uncircumcised

My penis is circumcised. Am I missing out on anything because I don't have my foreskin? – *Farid*

My penis is uncircumcised. Is it healthier to be circumcised?
– *Manoj*

It is estimated that approximately between 30–40 per cent of penis-owners globally are circumcised,[4] mainly in infancy or childhood, for religious or cultural reasons.

Some studies suggest that the foreskin may contribute somewhat to the experience of sexual pleasure. On the other hand, circumcision does have certain health benefits: it has been found to lower the risk of contracting sexually transmitted infections, including HIV, and can make it easier to keep the penis clean.

My two cents when it comes to penises is that it doesn't really matter all that much whether one is circumcised or not.

While some people feel it's not fair to make a decision about a person's body for them when they are a child and have no say in the matter, and therefore advocate against circumcision, it is a procedure that is easier and safer if performed in infancy—so the 'morality' of circumcision for cultural reasons for penis owners, remains a topic of heated debate.

Some people may require circumcision as adults for medical reasons, such as phimosis.

---

4 'Estimation of Country-specific and Global Prevalence of Male Circumcision', Brian J. Morris, Richard G. Wamai, Esther B. Henebeng, Aaron A.R. Tobian, Jeffrey D. Klausner, Joya Banerjee and Catherine A. Hankins, https://pophealthmetrics.biomedcentral.com/articles/10.1186/s12963-016-0073-5

Aesthetically, neither circumcised nor uncircumcised 'looks better' than the other. They just look a little different from each other.

In an uncircumcised penis, the foreskin is present, while in a circumcised penis, it has been removed—that's all!

Phimosis

My foreskin is so tight, it hurts during sex! What's going on? – *Nisham*

In an uncircumcised penis, the foreskin can typically slide over the penis, covering and uncovering the head or glans. However, if the foreskin is too tight, it may be unable to move this way. This condition is called **phimosis**: it's when the foreskin is too tight to be pulled back over the head or glans of the penis.

Children are born with tight foreskin. Most uncircumcised babies and toddlers will have phimosis, meaning the foreskin cannot be retracted. This is because the glans and the foreskin remain connected for the first few years of life. It's usually not a cause for concern in early childhood as the foreskin simply becomes retractable over time.

In adults, there are a number of risk factors and causes of phimosis, such as certain skin conditions, infections and balanitis, or inflammation of the glans.

Treatment for phimosis depends on the severity of the condition.

If phimosis interferes with your erections or urination, or if you experience any pain, swelling, bleeding or discomfort, you should see a doctor. Treatment exists. Topical treatments may be suggested for minor cases of phimosis, while adult circumcision may be required in more severe cases.

Morning Erections

I often wake up with an erection. Should I be worried? – *Rizwan*

Most people with penises will have experienced waking up in the morning with an erection. The slang term for this is **morning wood** and, hopefully, at this point, you'll have already guessed what I'm going to say next: it's totally normal!

The technical term for this is **nocturnal penile tumescence** or NPT. It's not something to worry about—it's just a function of the reproductive system and indicates that the nerves and blood supply to the penis are healthy.

Morning erections or NPT need not indicate sexual arousal or a sex dream—it is just the result of the sleep cycle combined with healthy nerves and blood flow in the body. The erection usually subsides soon after you wake up.

The frequency of NPT can vary from person to person based on things like age, hormones and health conditions. It is common for young people to experience this very often, and the frequency may decline with age.

And, guess what, morning erections can happen to people with vulvas too. Remember, early on in the book, we went over the fact that the clitoris and the penis develop from the same foetal tissue and share many similarities? Yup! It's less visibly obvious given that the clitoris tends to be much smaller than the penis to begin with, but you can wake up with an erect clitoris for similar reasons, and it's totally fine. It's just the body doing its thing, and the erection subsides soon!

Erectile Dysfunction

A woman once reached out to me to tell me the story of how **erectile dysfunction** (ED) sabotaged a burgeoning romance—but not for the reasons you might think.

She had developed feelings for a man she'd met online, and was really looking forward to having sex with him. But whenever the opportunity arose, he seemed to have trouble achieving an erection. And while she wanted to be empathetic and supportive by acknowledging that erectile dysfunction is a common, treatable issue, he became angry and rude when she mentioned that he could seek professional help and then refused to communicate with her thereafter.

She was heartbroken because she really liked him and would have been happy to support him while he figured this out. But after she brought up the idea that he may perhaps have a sexual health issue and should see a doctor, he abruptly ended the relationship.

She reached out to me to share her story in the hope that other people going through this might be spared the shame and heartbreak and, instead, embrace rather than push away a partner trying to be supportive.

So what exactly is erectile dysfunction?

Some people have difficulty achieving or maintaining an erection. In fact, this is more common than most of us might think. Erectile dysfunction is *extremely common* and yet many penis owners feel too embarrassed or ashamed to see a doctor because of the deep-rooted shame around not being able to 'perform' sexually and the prevalent associations of masculinity with sexual prowess and the like.

While pop culture can make it seem like men should always be ready for sex, it's normal not to feel sexual *all the time*, no matter your gender. Many penis-owners will have experienced variations in their ability to achieve or maintain an erection even if they don't have erectile dysfunction.

Stress, alcohol, medication and even just not being in the mood—these can all impact your ability to have an erection. And that's okay.

However, if you regularly find it difficult getting or keeping a firm enough erection to be able to have penetrative sex, it is possible that you might have erectile dysfunction. The good news is, it is a treatable condition. So it's certainly worth seeing a doctor.

Here's what's actually going on physiologically when someone gets an erection: the blood vessels in the penis relax and open up, allowing blood to fill them. This makes the penis 'hard'.

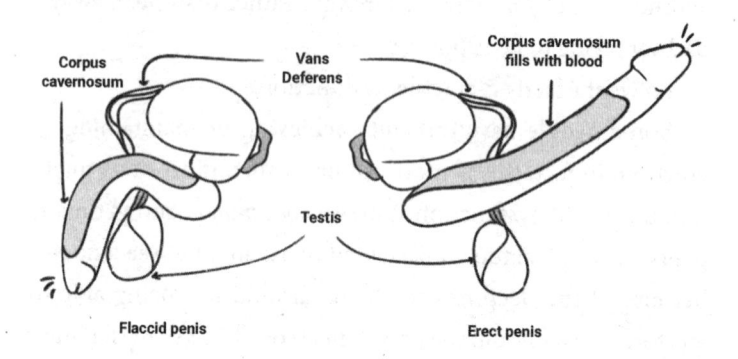

Corpus cavernosum • Vans Deferens • Corpus cavernosum fills with blood • Testis

Flaccid penis — Erect penis

Thus common physical causes of erectile dysfunction are related to blood circulation and blood pressure. For example, heart disease, atherosclerosis, high cholesterol and high blood pressure can all impact the amount of blood flowing to the penis and thereby contribute to ED.

On the other hand, ED can also be rooted in psychological issues—especially in people under forty. For example, mental health conditions like depression or anxiety can impact your libido, and even stress can make erections more difficult. After all, *arousal begins in the brain.*

It's worth overcoming any feelings of embarrassment and realizing that ED can happen to anyone, and that it can be treated with medication, therapy, exercises, and more. There's no shame in seeking help!

And whether or not ED is a concern for you, here's my top tip for penis-owners who want to do more to ensure their partner's pleasure: open your mind to the possibility of adding a sex toy to the mix during partnered play (with their consent, of course). The technology exists, and it's extremely effective, so why are we so reluctant to use it?

A vibrator and/or dildo is not your competition; it can be your best conspirator. What a *wonderfully* fun way to enhance your partner's pleasure while easing yourself of all that anxiety-inducing 'performance pressure'.

Why do I struggle to get an erection after I've had a few drinks? – *Dhruva*

Alcohol can meddle with the body's ability to get or maintain an erection. The phenomenon of being unable to get it up after having too much to drink is extremely common—so much so, that in slang terms it's called 'whiskey dick' or 'brewers droop'.

Many people think of alcohol as something that helps them shed their inhibitions—and so combining alcohol and sex is pretty common. But it's worth keeping in mind that alcohol can impair both your thinking and your bodily functioning. It can become difficult or even impossible to navigate consent when you're drunk, and as with whiskey dick—it can also make it hard to get hard.

Q Is masturbation bad for me and my penis?

I receive scores of messages every day from young men concerned about whether masturbation can harm their health, their penises or their relationships.

Will masturbation shrink my penis? Make it bigger? Reduce my sperm count? Can masturbation cause acne? Hair fall? Blindness? Hairy palms? Is masturbating while in a relationship equivalent to cheating? Will I go to hell because I masturbate?

The answer to all these questions is a resounding NO!

In fact, masturbation is the safest way one can experience sexual pleasure—without the risks of infection or pregnancy. It is a perfectly normal, self-soothing behaviour and can even have several health benefits including stress relief and better sleep. If you don't like to masturbate, that's fine too—but there's nothing inherently bad or wrong about it and it cannot cause any of the problems listed above.

A lot of people feel guilty about masturbating and therefore feel afraid that 'bad things' will happen to them because they masturbate. Often parents, teachers, religious leaders and the like spout unscientific ideas to scare people and shame them when it comes to anything to do with sexual pleasure—so we tend to inherit a lot of shame around masturbation. That might result in feelings of guilt or fear around the act and a tendency to associate masturbation with actually unrelated 'negative outcomes'—that's certainly something to think about too.

For example, if you think masturbation is bad for you, you're more likely to assume that the pimple you got today was because you masturbated yesterday when, actually, that's just a coincidence—there's no causal link between the two. *Overcoming those feelings of guilt and shame is likely to result in a more comfortable relationship with your body.*

How often is it okay to masturbate? I masturbate almost every day, sometimes 2–3 times a day, and usually I also watch porn. Do I masturbate too much? – *Tejas*

Some people may masturbate daily, some may do it a few times a month, others maybe masturbate once a week—there's no 'right' amount and it's also okay not to do it at all. You get to decide.

However, if you feel that masturbating is getting in the way of school, work or family commitments, then maybe you want to think about it.

If your genitals are literally chafing from too much friction or you're starting to feel like you simply cannot do without masturbating, then, like any other behaviour you may feel a lack of control over—for me it's my screen time and use of Instagram—you might want to think of cutting back.

Another reason so many people and, more specifically, many men, seem to worry that masturbation is a problem is perhaps because in the internet era, porn and masturbation are often bucketed together. And because a lot of mainstream porn is hugely problematic in how it's produced and how it depicts things like gender roles and race, masturbation also gets a negative image along with porn, when in fact, masturbation is actually pretty good for you—it's the mainstream porn that has the issues.

Even the controversial No-Fap movement in fact came up primarily in response to mainstream internet porn and concerns around the possibility of 'porn addiction', not the act of masturbation itself.

Masturbation can be a helpful, safe way to experience sexual release, explore your sexuality, understand your body better, and figure out what feels good for you. Some studies even suggest that masturbation can reduce period cramps for people who menstruate and may even reduce the risk of prostate cancer for people with prostates.

So here's my take: whatever your gender, *don't feel bad or guilty about masturbating*. It isn't inherently harmful. Celebrate yourself and savour your body's capacity for pleasure.

As with anything else in life, it's just worth being mindful if you ever begin to feel like something is making you act compulsively. I, for example, love using social media, but I do sometimes feel that endless scrolling can get in the way of my ability to focus on other things. If you feel like something is getting in the way of your ability to function in your daily life, you can think about cutting back on that activity or taking a break so that you can re-establish a healthy relationship with that thing.

And let's not forget that it is possible to masturbate without porn. Try it sometime!

BALLS: THE TESTES AND SCROTUM

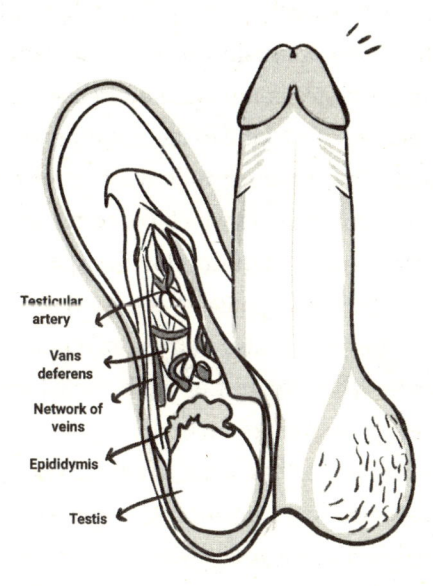

Labels on diagram: Testicular artery, Vans deferens, Network of veins, Epididymis, Testis

One of my balls is a bit bigger than the other. Is this normal?
– *Sid*

Should I be concerned that one of my balls seems positioned slightly lower than the other? – *Abhimanyu*

Below the penis, surrounded by pubic hair, are the **testicles** or **balls**. These are a pair of oval-shaped organs located together in a single sac called the scrotum, or ball sac.

The testes have two main functions: to produce sperm and to produce hormones, particularly **testosterone**. They can also be a source of pleasure during sexual activity.

The testes grow in size during puberty. It's common for one testicle to be slightly bigger or hang slightly lower than the other—these are not usually causes for concern.

Each of the testes comprises hundreds of metres of small, coiled tubes, which are kind of like a subway system for sperm. After puberty, they produce millions of sperm every day.

The **scrotum** or **sac** in which the testes are encased is like temperature-regulated housing for the sperm factory. While the fact that they hang outside the body makes them more vulnerable to injury, it also allows for them to remain a few degrees cooler than the rest of the body, which is thought to assist in healthy sperm production.

The scrotum also has some amount of elasticity, so it can bring your testes closer to your body when you're cold and lets them hang lower when you're warm.

The skin that the scrotum is made of is very similar to the skin that comprises the inner labial folds of people with vulvas.

Q What's the difference between sperm and semen?

Many of us think of semen and sperm as synonyms—but, in fact, they're not exactly the same.

Sperm are the tiny tadpole-shaped cells produced by the testes that are central to reproduction. Sperm can fertilize an egg to cause a pregnancy.

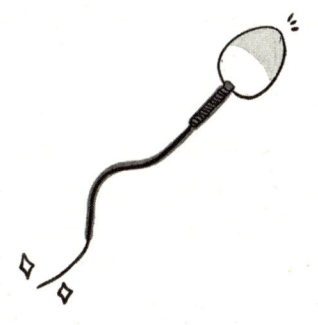

But you can't actually *see* sperm without a microscope. What you see is called semen—the whitish fluid that is produced by the seminal vesicles to help transport the sperm out of the penis during ejaculation.

Semen exits the penis via the same canal that urine comes out of—the urethra. But not to worry, you cannot both ejaculate and pee simultaneously—the mechanism only allows either one or the other fluid to exit at a time.

And while semen typically does contain sperm, **not all sperm ends up as semen**.

The body produces millions of sperm every day that doesn't necessarily exit the body as semen—if ejaculation doesn't take place, sperm is simply reabsorbed by the body.

The body has its own mechanisms for discarding and recycling unused/dead cells—and sperm cells are no different in this regard. Unused sperm is simply broken down by the body and new sperm is produced.

Likewise, **not all semen contains sperm**. People who have had a vasectomy or who have azoospermia may produce semen that has no sperm in it.

A **vasectomy** is a small surgical procedure performed on the *vas deferens* (the tube that transports sperm from the testes to the urethra so it can exit the penis with semen during ejaculation). A vasectomy blocks the sperm from reaching the semen. It is one of the most effective forms of contraception. People who have had a vasectomy produce semen that does not have sperm in it.

Azoospermia is a condition where the semen of a penis-owner does not contain sperm because the testicles are unable to properly make or transport sperm. There are a number of different potential causes, such as a blockage, certain injuries, infections or health conditions. However, this condition is relatively rare.

Q What is precum?

Precum is a small amount of clear liquid that can come out of the penis when you're aroused—it's not the same as semen or cum. It's often released considerably before ejaculation takes place, hence the name *pre* cum. It can act as a sort of natural lubricant similar to the way the vagina may release lubrication and get wet when aroused. You can't control precum—it may or may not happen, but either way it's involuntary.

Q Can you get pregnant from precum?

Precum can potentially contain sperm which is one of the reasons why it's important to use protection from the get-go rather than putting on a condom later or opting to pull out only

Nightfall

Sometimes, while asleep, in the middle of the night, semen seems to come out of my penis. Is this normal? – *Jai*

Nocturnal emission or **nightfall**, colloquially called a '**wet dream**', is a spontaneous or involuntary orgasm that occurs during sleep. Essentially, it consists of ejaculation for penis-owners or vaginal lubrication for people with vaginas (yes it does happen to us too!).

Nightfall doesn't happen only at night. You could have a wet dream even if you're sleeping during the day. And since we're talking terminology, wet 'dream' is a bit of a misnomer too because it may or may not be accompanied by an actual dream.

Wet dreams may occur for anyone of any gender, at any point in life after puberty. Which is why sometimes you may wake up to find your pyjamas or sheets a little wet.

It's simply more common during adolescence or during periods of sexual abstinence. It's totally normal and shouldn't be viewed as bad or wrong.

A natural and involuntary occurrence, nightfall in no way compromises your health or sexual functioning. In fact, it is so common that most people will have experienced a wet dream at some point in their lives.

That said, it is also totally okay not to have them. Many people experience wet dreams, but some people don't. And since this is stuff we rarely ever talk about or get educated about, many people may also have had wet dreams without acknowledging or realizing it.

Our bodies are incredible organisms, and so many of even the most important functions they perform—from our heartbeat to breathing to digestion—are all involuntary. The body often just does its own thing. It's meant to. Wet dreams or nightfall are just one more thing that it does sometimes. It is a perfectly natural occurrence and nothing to be concerned about.

There are also several misconceptions about wet dreams that I'd like to quickly clear up. A wet dream is not you peeing in your sleep. A wet dream does not reduce sperm count. It is not a sign of illness. It does not shrink the penis. And it isn't sinful or bad or dirty or something to be ashamed of or feel guilty about. At the most, you might have to change your pyjamas or wash your sheets!

Premature Ejaculation

I cum pretty quickly—should I be concerned about premature ejaculation? – *Simon*

My partner and I are unable to climax at the same time. I almost always cum before she does. What can I do to last longer in bed? – *Virendra*

Premature ejaculation (PE) is when a person with a penis frequently or always ejaculates sooner than they would like. PE is an extremely common concern among penis-owners.

While you can see a urologist and/or sex therapist about PE if you like, here are some things to keep in mind:

You can probably complete my sentence for me at this point, but **sex is more than just penetration!**

Also, simultaneous orgasms are kind of rare—most couples don't climax at exactly the same time! In fact, that mostly happens only in the movies.

Instead, keep in mind that sex doesn't have to end just because the person with the penis ejaculated. You can take turns pleasuring each other.

Here are some ideas if you'd like to explore how you can 'last longer':

Slow things down instead of speeding things up—spend a lot of time on the acts considered 'foreplay': kissing, oral sex, manual stimulation, massages, cuddling, playing with the breasts and nipples, or the thighs and butt.

Try **edging**—also called the 'start-stop' technique. Pausing each time you feel you're getting close to ejaculation, and then resuming till you need to pause again. Doing this a few times before you ejaculate can help you prolong the time till climax as well as build to an extra-exciting orgasm.

And instead of focusing only on the genitals, enjoy the less obvious spots too—tickling, licking, or even just breathing on body parts like your partner's ears, neck, back, or behind their knees, or caressing their hair or even their feet—can also provide surprisingly intense pleasure and prolong intimacy while still keeping everyone extremely aroused.

Q What is the refractory period?

Why can't I keep going after I ejaculate? Why do I need to take a break after I cum, before I can have sex or cum again?
– *Neil*

For penis-owners usually after sexual stimulation that results in orgasm and ejaculation, there's a brief period during which the body won't respond to further sexual stimulation. This is called the refractory period. It's a sort of recovery or resolution period during which the body slowly returns to its normal level of functioning. The penis usually becomes flaccid, and you might sort of just feel like you need a breather for a few minutes, or hours.

It's unlikely you'll be able to experience erection or ejaculation for a little while as you've just experienced it and your body needs a moment to rest before it can get started again.

While some vulva-owners may also feel like they need a breather after an orgasm, or might not be in the mood for more sex, physiologically, vulva-owners are often able to continue to respond to sexual stimulation and have multiple orgasms, whereas penis-owners are likely to need some time before the penis is able to experience erection and ejaculation again once they have cum.

The duration of the refractory period varies among individuals and can change with age.

Blue Balls

If I don't ejaculate by masturbating or having sex when I'm aroused or erect, will it be bad for my health or my penis?
– *Madhav*

My boyfriend says he'll get 'blue balls' if we don't have sex when he's aroused. Is this true? Do I have to have sex with him because of this? – *Sakshi*

People mistakenly see sexual arousal as some sort of necessary call to action. This is especially common in the way that male sexuality and the penis are talked about, but it's a rather silly and harmful idea. Literally nothing will happen to your health if you just let those feelings subside.

The phenomenon of 'blue balls' and, in fact, by the same logic, even 'blue vulvas', is simply an expression to describe the fact that the genitals become engorged with blood when aroused, and this can even lend them a slightly darker hue temporarily thanks to the extra blood supply. It's nothing to worry about and subsides on its own.

Not acting on arousal does not compromise one's health or the health and function of the genitals, and 'blue balls' is not a valid reason to persuade a partner to have sex.

In fact, *I don't think there's a single valid reason to try to 'persuade' someone to have sex against their will. Don't do it. Sex should always be something both partners genuinely want to experience together. It's not something you should coax someone to do for you if they don't want it.*

Delayed Ejaculation

I take forever to ejaculate. I know that sounds like I'm bragging, but trust me, just like premature ejaculation is a problem, even this is a problem. I usually can't manage to come long after my girlfriend has finished. It's very awkward, and after 30–40 minutes sometimes it still doesn't happen, both of us are tired, and I'm left feeling embarrassed and inadequate. Even though I've tried to explain it's an issue I have, I think my girlfriend takes it personally or something, and worries there's something I don't like about her—because the men she'd been with previously would come pretty quickly. Can you please talk about delayed ejaculation so more people realize it is genuinely a condition some people face? – *Umesh*

Indeed, some people may experience delayed ejaculation—which is when ejaculation takes a very long time to occur despite sufficient stimulation to the penis, or when ejaculation does not occur at all (also called anejaculation). It may be lifelong or acquired; and it may be general or situational. It may result from physical factors such as chronic health conditions, medications, or surgeries; substance misuse or overuse; and/or psychological factors such as depression, anxiety, stress, past trauma, poor body image and insecurities about performance.

Treatment may include prescribing certain medications, or revising your current medication intake, if you're on medication that could be causing the issue. Psychological counselling can help any underlying mental health concerns.

While it can be awkward and frustrating to experience delayed ejaculation because of how conditioned we are to see ejaculation as some sort of cornerstone of sex, it's worth remembering that sex doesn't always have to end in ejaculation for it to be pleasurable. Don't feel like you can't stop until you ejaculate. Stop when you both want to stop.

THE PROSTATE: AN EROGENOUS ZONE MANY DON'T KNOW ABOUT!

The prostate, sometimes referred to as the 'P-spot' or the 'male G-spot', is a gland located between the bladder and the penis, which can be stimulated via the anus.

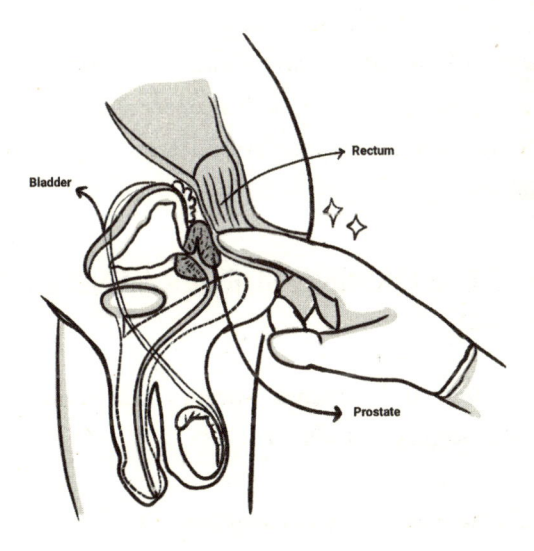

The prostate's main function is to produce fluid that makes up semen—but it can also be a source of intense pleasure.

While you can access the prostate via the anus using fingers, penetration, **pegging**, or toys like **prostate massagers** and **butt plugs** (see page 218), it can also be stimulated by externally massaging the perineum—the area between the anus and the penis.

I'm not a big fan of the term 'male G-spot' to refer to the prostate because, by association, it suggests the existence of the 'female' G-spot which is in fact not a gland or structure at all but simply an erogenous zone for vagina-owners. Also, all people with prostates don't necessarily identify as men, just as all people with vaginas don't necessarily identify as women.

Still, since this is a phrase commonly used to refer to the prostate, I wanted to clarify that P-Spot, 'male G-spot' and prostate all refer to the same thing.

People of any sexual orientation can explore and enjoy prostate stimulation solo or with a consenting partner. It is not something that is determined by or determining of your sexual orientation.

GENDER-AFFIRMING SURGERY AND THE GENITALS

What is 'top' and 'bottom' surgery and what is gender affirming surgery? – *Karuna*

What is a neopenis and a neovagina? – *Lalita*

What exactly is gender dysphoria? – *Dee*

Gender dysphoria is feelings of distress or unease caused by a sense of dissonance between one's gender identity and one's sex assigned at birth.

Many trans people report experiencing dysphoria, and some may choose to explore gender-affirming services and interventions: via dressing and bodily self-expression, such as transfeminine folks 'tucking' the penis and/or wearing 'femme' clothing, hair and makeup; or transmasculine folks 'binding' the chest and cultivating a 'masc' appearance; and/or medical interventions such as hormone therapy and **gender-affirming surgery**.

The gender-affirmation process is unique to each person—and it may or may not involve surgery. Some people may seek surgery as part of their transition while others may not. There is no single, 'right' way to be trans, just as there is no single, 'right' way to be human.

Gender-affirming surgery can include **top surgery** and/or **bottom surgery**. Top surgery generally entails the removal or construction of breasts, while bottom surgery generally involves the creation of external genitals that affirm one's gender identity, and/or the removal of internal reproductive organs.

For transfeminine people who opt for gender-affirming surgery, procedures may include placing breast implants and/or orchiectomy (removal of the testes) and/or vaginoplasty and/or vulvoplasty, where a vaginal canal and/or vulva may be constructed. There are several different types of vaginoplasty and vulvoplasty procedures which use different types of skin and tissue differently, but often penile and scrotal tissue is used to construct a **neovagina** (a vagina that is constructed through surgery). A good surgeon will prioritize pleasure and sensation such that a neovagina is capable of both clitoral and vaginal sensation and orgasm. For example, a clitoris may be created using a portion of the head of the penis, and the prostate may serve as an internal erogenous zone similar to the G-spot.

A neovagina may require slightly different practices in terms of care and hygiene than a natal vagina (a vagina someone is born with). For example, neovaginas are sometimes not self-cleaning and so can be cleaned with mild soap and water. Depending on the type of skin used to create the vaginal canal during surgery, a neovagina may or may not be self-lubricating; it may also require dilation.

For transmasculine people who opt for gender-affirming surgery, procedures may include mastectomy (removal of the breasts), and/or hysterectomy (removal of the uterus) and/or vaginectomy (removal of the vagina) and/or metoidioplasty or phalloplasty (construction of a penis). Just as a surgically constructed vagina is sometimes referred to as a neovagina in medical contexts, a surgically constructed penis may be called a **neopenis**. In a metoidioplasty, the clitoris is transformed into a neopenis, while in a phalloplasty, skin grafted from the arm, thigh, back or abdomen is typically used. A scrotoplasty—the creation of a scrotum—is sometimes undergone alongside a metoidioplasty or phalloplasty. In a scrotoplasty, the labia majora is repositioned and hollowed out to form a scrotum, and silicone testicular implants may be inserted. Preserving sexual sensation can be prioritized such that people can continue to experience pleasure and orgasm after genital reconstruction procedures.

In the words of @trintrin (Dr Trinetra Haldar Gummaraju), whom you absolutely must follow on Instagram if you aren't already, we must 'realize that trans women are women, and trans men are men, irrespective of medical intervention. Non-binary trans people are non-binary irrespective of medical intervention too. Acknowledge and respect identity.'

Among her story highlights, where you'll find deeply informative and thought-provoking meditations on gender and sexuality as well as about her own transition, I discovered these beautiful lines from an absolutely gorgeous poem called 'How to Make Love to a Transperson' by Gabe Moses:

Realize that bodies are only a fraction of who we are
They're just oddly-shaped vessels for hearts
And honestly, they can barely contain us
We strain at their seams with every breath we take
We are all pulse and sweat,
Tissue and nerve ending
We are programmed to grope and fumble until we get it right.
Bodies have been learning each other forever.
It's what bodies do.
They are grab bags of parts
And half the fun is figuring out
All the different ways we can fit them together;
All the different uses for hipbones and hands,

Tongues and teeth;
All the ways to car-crash our bodies beautiful.
But we could never forget how to use our hearts
Even if we tried.
That's the important part.
Don't worry about the bodies.
They've got this.

Don't worry about the bodies. They've got this.

BOUNDARIES

As I conclude this section on anatomy, I'd like to remind you that unless you're someone's lover or their doctor, and only if you've already established that it's a topic you are both comfortable discussing, please don't comment on or ask people questions about their genitals or body.

People frequently send me questions like: 'What's your boob size?' 'Do you have a protruding or tucked-in labia?'

Queer and trans people, and people with disabilities, are often asked even more ridiculous, rude and invasive questions about their bodies.

Don't be that person who has no boundaries. Not on the internet, not in real life. No one owes you any explanations about their bodies. And one's genitals are no one else's business but one's own.

Sex

*What You Need to Know
Long Before You Get Naked*

FIRST SEXUAL EXPERIENCES

I'm 17 and I'm thinking of having sex with my girlfriend (same age). Do you think we are too young? – *Prateek*

I'm 28 and I'm embarrassed to admit that I've never had sex. Is it too late? – *Trina*

Q What is the 'right' age to have sex?

This is a question without an easy answer.

Age of consent laws vary widely across the world. To give you a sense of how drastically they can differ across countries, here are some examples:[5]

In Bahrain, the legal age of consent is twenty-one. It is the country with the highest age of consent. In India, Turkey, Argentina, and several other countries, the age of consent is eighteen. In most states in the US, as well as in Canada, the UK, Russia, Australia, and several others, it is sixteen. In countries including Thailand, Cambodia, Denmark, Sweden and Costa

---

5 'Ages of Consent around the World', *The Week*, UK, https://www.theweek.co.uk/92121/ages-of-consent-around-the-world

Rica, it is fifteen. In Germany, Italy, China and Brazil, among others, it is fourteen. In Japan, and a few other countries, it is thirteen. In Angola, it is twelve.

In many countries, primarily in North Africa and the Middle East, including Afghanistan, Iran, Saudi Arabia, the UAE, Kuwait, Oman, Qatar, Sudan and Libya, as well as Pakistan, the Maldives, and others, sexual activity is illegal before or outside of marriage.

In many countries where sex without marriage is illegal, the minimum age of marriage is lower for women than for men. And in several countries, it remains common for courts to grant permission to girls to marry below the legal age. In India too, even though child marriage is illegal, it still takes place.

Societies and their lawmakers globally clearly do not share a consensus on what the 'right' minimum legal age of consent to sex should be. And the fact that in several countries these laws have been amended over time indicates the ways in which perspectives on sexual and bodily autonomy and gender equality have evolved across history and in different geographies.

For example, under the Indian Penal Code, in 1860, the age of consent was only for 'girls' and was initially ten years of age. This was raised to twelve in 1891, fourteen in 1925, sixteen in 1940 and eighteen in 2013. In South Korea, the age of consent was thirteen till 2020—it is now sixteen.

In these and many other 'developing' countries, raising the age of consent has been seen as a progressive step in the interest of the rights of women and children. Yet, for example, as I mentioned, in several western European and Scandinavian countries—like Germany, Denmark and Sweden, considered the pinnacles of the 'developed' world—the age of consent has long been, and remains, fourteen or fifteen.

As I said, the question of what is the 'right' age by which people should be able to have sex, even legally, has no single easy answer. Lawmakers globally have the challenge of having to determine how they can protect the safety and rights of young people without infringing on their agency and autonomy.

I am of the opinion that we need to have different laws for sexual activity between consenting teenagers, and different laws for sexual activity between adults and minors.

Child marriage and forced marriages should have no place in our world. And laws need to protect children, adolescents and teenagers from sexual or emotional abuse by adults.

On the other hand, consensual sex between older teenagers similar in age appears to be an inevitability, globally, and we should empower young people with the information and resources they need to ensure that they can make safer, better choices around their health and well-being. Young people deserve access to comprehensive sex education, consent training, contraception, STI testing and treatment, and safe abortion services.

As is evident in the contrast between Prateek and Trina's messages at the top of this section, while a lot of the concern around the 'right age' for sex is oriented around people having sex 'too young', paradoxically, society also leaves some people feeling rather anxious or embarrassed about not having had sex by a certain age.

There is no rush to have sex. And it's okay not to have had sex, whatever your age.

In India, where most people live with their families well into adulthood, privacy is a scarce commodity, and our relationships tend to be closely surveilled by family members, if we are allowed to have relationships before marriage at all. More people than you might imagine have sex for the first time in their twenties or later.

As an adult, it really ought to be up to you to decide if and when you are ready to explore a sexual relationship.

Q What is sex like the first time?

Like with anything you're doing for the first time, the idea of your first sexual experience can seem exciting, confusing, scary, or all of the above.

On top of that, sex is rarely talked about.

So a lot of us coming into our first sexual experiences don't know enough about consent, contraception, safety or pleasure.

Sex does come with the risk of outcomes like accidental pregnancy and infection, and it's worth understanding this so you can do your best to mitigate these risks by adopting safer sexual practices.

Only barrier methods like condoms help protect against **both** pregnancy and infection. So, as far as protection goes, they are your best bet for first-time sex. They are easily available, relatively cheap, and can provide contraception, as well as protection against STI transmission during vaginal, oral and anal sex.

Still, it's worth understanding that no method of protection can ever be 100 per cent safe. Human error or contraceptive failure can occur, and both unplanned pregnancies and sexually transmitted infections are far more common than most people think—so it's also really worth figuring out for yourself beforehand what you would do were you to find yourself in such a situation.

Identifying a trustworthy and competent gynaecologist/ andrologist in your vicinity that you can consult is one of the most useful things you can do for yourself as an adult.

I will elaborate on contraception and STI prevention and treatment in the section on safety (see page 124). So for now, let's get back to discussing the sort of headspace most of us bring to our first sexual experiences.

We've typically already internalized some garbage expectations and pressures around sex at this point—maybe there's pressure to have sex to seem 'cool', maybe there's pressure not to have sex to stay 'pure'.

There are also ideas that we internalize around gender and sex that I've already outlined over the course of this book—we're made to believe that men should always want it and that women should not, that men are entitled to it and that women are obligated to provide it.

There's also far too little mainstream public dialogue and representation around queer identity and queer sexual experiences.

For many of us, coming into our early sexual experiences, we tend to think that having sex is necessarily the act of a penis in a vagina, that non-penetrative sexual activity is somehow less legitimate.

This penetration-centric view of sex perpetuates the idea that only heterosexual vaginal intercourse is sex as well as the problematic construct of 'virginity' which posits women as passive recipients—she 'gives' her virginity, he 'takes' it.

Consider, also, phrases like 'deflower', 'pop her cherry', or 'seal todna'—in describing the stakes for a woman having intercourse for the first time.

Not only do these bear the weight of the damaging and unscientific 'hymen myth' I've explained in the section on the anatomy of the vulva (see page 18), they also suggest the idea that women's bodies are a site of 'conquest', where they 'lose' something, while the man 'wins' something during sex and, particularly, first-time sex.

There's an undertone of violence and shame attached to the phrases, as also to many other phrases used to describe sex in this type of gendered manner—as if the man's role is necessarily that of an aggressor or predator and the woman's, that of a victim or gatekeeper.

If penetration was instead called 'envelopment', for example, or 'losing your virginity' was instead phrased 'making your sexual debut,' wouldn't we see it all a bit differently?

And as I mentioned, this heteronormative, penetration-centric view of 'sex' and 'virginity' also de-legitimizes queer sex: some people's sexual experiences may never entail a penis in a vagina, and those are still absolutely legitimate sexual experiences.

Isn't it rather sad that this heteronormative and misogynistic view of sex remains the dominant paradigm we inherit within which we develop our perspective on sex and sexuality, colouring our expectations and imagination, even before we've ever had a sexual experience of our own?

Sex can be whatever you and your partner want it to be. Oral sex is sex, anal sex is sex... mutual masturbation, outercourse, using a sex toy, using your hands—all this, and more, can be sex. And the idea that having sex for the first time is some sort of 'loss', as in the phrase 'losing' your virginity, is one we're best off discarding.

Whatever your gender identity and sexual orientation, sex stands to be a wonderful, equal, shared expression and experience of things like desire, intimacy, attraction, trust, vulnerability, joy, pleasure, love, and so much more—it can encompass a whole range of physical and emotional possibilities.

But as with doing most things for the first time, often the first time is a learning experience—things may feel a little bit clumsy or awkward, and that's okay.

It can be a meaningful experience, or at the very least, a sweet and fun experience, if you're both kind and respectful of each other and go into it with a sense of empathy and non-judgmental curiosity.

But it's also okay to feel underwhelmed. Many people find first-time sex to feel like less of a big deal than they thought it would be.

Particularly for vulva-owners, given how little young people are taught about the vulva in relation to pleasure, first sexual experiences are often kind of, well, anticlimactic, if we're honest.

However, first-time sex should not hurt. Sex isn't meant to be inherently painful—we need to get rid of the myth that pain is just a part of the sexual experience; that idea is harmful and untrue.

Pain is usually the result of insufficient lubrication, insufficient 'foreplay', an injury, or a health condition—as I've explained in the section on the body (see page 42).

Don't do anything that hurts. It may even take several attempts at vaginal or anal sex before you're able to 'go all the way' comfortably, and that's okay.

Use lube, go slow, be gentle with each other, communicate, take your time.

When it comes to understanding one another's body and pleasure, it's likely that the first time won't be the 'best' time. But it's also very likely that you will get better at it as you go along. And what a fun journey that can be, exploring and celebrating the body—pleasure can be a lifelong learning experience.

What we all certainly can and should work at learning about long before we start having sex, though, is consent.

CONSENT

What is consent, exactly? I know people say it's important to understand when someone says no, or that only an enthusiastic yes means you want to go ahead with something, but I find it really hard to communicate my needs and preferences honestly with partners, both inside and outside the bedroom. I often feel confused and tongue-tied, both when I want to initiate or express something, as well as when I don't feel like doing something they want to do. It's like I'm somehow not able to say what I mean, because this stuff just feels really difficult and awkward to talk about, especially whenever I'm dating someone new. Also, sometimes I think I'm not entirely sure what I want. How can we get better at talking about our feelings, even our mixed feelings? Isn't it actually pretty hard, or am I just inept? – *Tithi*

'Yes', 'No', and Beyond

In theory, consent can sound like the most basic idea in the world: the dictionary definition is simply 'to give permission for something to happen; agreement to do something'. But in practice, and particularly in the context of sexual interactions, it can certainly be tricky to navigate.

Slogans intended to clarify the idea of consent have ranged from 'no means no' to 'only yes means yes', and sex educators, including myself, routinely pronounce that consent needs to be 'enthusiastic'.

And while these sorts of pithy one-line catchphrases are well-meaning and can be helpful, I want to acknowledge that the challenges that are posed by the complex terrain of consent can extend far beyond their purview.

'No means no' makes the assumption that people are unanimously able to turn down something they don't want to do. But we know that that is not always the case. Unfortunately, it is sometimes neither easy, safe, or even possible, to say no.

Most of us will have at some point felt pressured to agree to do things we don't actually want to do, whether in a sexual or non-sexual context, because we fear we'll be harmed or judged if we don't comply, or because we don't want to hurt the other person's feelings.

And, if we're honest, we've likely also been on the other side, even if unwittingly—where someone else agreed to do something we wanted to do even though they didn't really want to do it.

'Only yes means yes' tries to mitigate these issues by suggesting that a more affirmative approach might serve us better—the idea is that it is important to pay attention to how someone communicates even when they don't explicitly say 'no', and that nothing other than an enthusiastic 'yes' signals consent.

This is helpful in that when someone says nothing, or seems reluctant, we should assume we do *not* have their consent, not assume that we do.

But even the 'only yes means yes' model eventually encounters the same pitfalls as the 'no means no' model.

Because if certain circumstances force people to say yes when they'd rather say no, even a seemingly enthusiastic yes cannot always imply a genuine willingness and eagerness to participate.

I myself have definitely been in more than one situation where I 'consented' to sex only because it seemed like the easiest way to exit the interaction safely or without hurting the other person's feelings. It is absolutely no fun to think about, but here we are.

While people of all genders may relate to this, it tends to be a majority experience for women.

'Why would you care about hurting the other person's feelings?!'

'If you don't want to do something, why don't you just say so and leave—slap them if necessary!'

Well-meaning folks have often said things like this to me with indignation when I have tried to broach the topic of just how frequently women end up having to do things with men that they would rather not do.

While it's tempting to think that consent violations including full-blown sexual assault are perpetrated only by monstrous strangers in dark alleyways, or a 'creep' one is meeting for the first time, the fact is that the majority of non-consensual sexual encounters and experiences of sexual violence actually take place with a perpetrator well-known to the person. Friends, acquaintances, family members, partners, spouses. Let's not forget that in 2022 marital rape is still legal in India.

On the flip side, I've also feigned reluctance to act on a desire even when in fact I would have been delighted to act on it, because I feared that if I gave in too quickly or too enthusiastically, they'd see me as 'easy'—surely a common fear in a society that so relentlessly slut-shames women and conditions us to see ourselves as sexual gatekeepers.

So how do we ensure that we can express ourselves both honestly and safely?

Paromita Vohra, the founder of the digital sex-education project, Agents of Ishq, and one of my favourite thinkers on all things relationships, sexuality and pleasure, created a wonderful Lavani, a traditional Maharashtrian dance performance, exploring consent (you can watch it on the Agents of Ishq YouTube channel), where she raises perhaps the most important yet under-addressed question of all: Can we make room for what lies in-between 'yes' and 'no' to also exist as we navigate consent? Can we make room to explore 'maybe' too?

We've *all* got to work on creating an environment of total honesty, respect, safety and kindness—where if, at any point, anyone feels that they don't really want to do something, we are not only able to but rather encouraged to communicate those feelings, whatever their nuance, without fear of consequence. *We need to collectively create a culture that values consent.*

Excitement, nervousness, hesitation, discomfort, fear, confusion—these are complex emotions that often present themselves during sexual encounters, and they can indeed be hard to immediately reduce to a definitive yes or no.

As human beings, surely the least we can do in our interactions is allow each other the time and space within which to figure out our emotions and feelings and desires safely, without the obligation of an immediate 'yes' or 'no' if we don't yet have an answer.

Instead of judging someone for saying no, or feeling anger, shame, or rejection when someone does not reciprocate our feelings or is unwilling to do something we want to, let's learn to feel gratitude that they are honouring their own boundaries and taking care of themselves.

And likewise, instead of judging someone for respectfully articulating their desires and seeming enthusiastic at the prospect of sex, let us allow each other the space to be vulnerable and honest about how we feel, without automatically also expecting or taking on the burden of reciprocation.

Doesn't asking for consent again and again just kill the mood though? – *Nakul*

I simply cannot buy the argument that actively seeking consent 'kills the mood'.

You know what most certainly will kill the mood? Violating someone's consent. By seeking rather than assuming consent, no matter how awkward you think you sound, you reduce the chances of participating in what you too, but certainly the other person, may reflect on as a highly negative and regrettable experience.

And if the person is indeed keen to participate with you, then seeking consent can serve almost as foreplay.

For most people, feeling safe and respected are prerequisites for being able to experience arousal. Talking about something before actually acting on the desire expressed can be incredibly sexy rather than a buzzkill!

To get better at navigating consent in our sexual relationships, we need to destigmatize talking about sex.

Part of the idea that discussing consent is awkward and 'ruins the moment' comes from the general overarching reluctance in a patriarchal, heteronormative, sex-negative world, to talk openly about anything to do with sex.

As a society, we refuse to talk about sex in general—so of course many find it awkward to actively, verbally approach consent too. For the awkwardness to dissipate we must also collectively normalize talking about sex.

The shame and silence and stigma around broaching sex as a topic of necessary public conversation makes it harder for people to navigate consent, to be assertive of their sexual preferences, to learn about pleasure, as well as to access sexual health services. It also protects perpetrators of sexual violence by making it difficult for survivors to speak up.

Together we need to cultivate a reciprocal attitude of respect and compassion within all human interactions. We need to establish that, in all contexts, but especially within sexual contexts, a willingness to honestly communicate our desires and curiosities and boundaries with one another is vital, and that the decision to perform a particular action in a partnered encounter cannot be made unilaterally.

To get better at navigating consent in our sexual relationships, we need to value consent in all aspects of life.

To create an overarching culture of consent in society, an understanding of and regard for consent needs to be cultivated long before our first sexual encounters. Our consent should absolutely matter in non-sexual contexts as well.

But many of us grow up having experienced indifference towards or, worse still, the ongoing and active dismissal of our own agency, autonomy and consent, well into adulthood.

From seemingly small things like forcing us to eat something we don't want to, or preventing us from wearing what we want to, to undeniably big things like forcing us to get married against our wishes, often to a person we didn't choose, many of us are raised in an environment with little regard for our consent—whether from family members, teachers, religious figures, bosses or other authority figures.

There's the domineering authority of the strict and often violent parent who requires you to always do as they say, no questions asked; there's the manipulative emotional blackmail of the overly doting parent that goads or guilts you into always doing things their way; there's the reverence for social mores over personal dreams—the notion that in any case it doesn't really matter what you want, what matters far more is *log kya kahenge*.

We need to do all we can to ensure that we do not perpetuate these behaviours from generation to generation. We have to be the change.

Consent Matters, No Matter Your Gender

Consent seems so important to you feminazis, soon men are going to have to bring a lawyer along to every date and draw up a contract before every hook-up. – *Rahul*

When I speak about consent on my digital platforms, a lot of disgruntled men leave snarky comments like this.

The agency and autonomy of women and queer people are disproportionately policed and targeted in both sexual and non-sexual contexts globally, and we desperately need to do better. But you aren't doing anyone any kind of big favour by simply being mindful of their consent. Seeking to understand and respect each other is the bare minimum human decency one can extend—no matter our gender.

Just as the narrative that women are sexual gatekeepers who only reluctantly participate in sex; that queer people and sexually confident women are 'asking for it'; and the absurd linkage of women's 'virginity' with their 'honour' is damaging and untrue, so also the narrative that men want sex all the time and that a 'real man' would never turn down sex is also damaging and untrue.

A lot of cishet men don't seem to grasp that a culture that disregards consent harms them too. Just as women who seem to want sex are 'sluts' while women who turn down sex are 'frigid', men who seem to want sex are 'creeps' while men who turn down sex are 'losers'. Do you see how broken the system is? There are no winners.

Consent as a Daily Practice

Consent is something all people deserve to be able to exercise without fear or shame. Consent needs to be *practised* by all parties. It is not a transaction. It is not something that is only 'given' or only 'received'. It is not a one-time action.

It is a practice, and in order to get better at it, *consent is something we need to be mindful about in every single interaction we have.*

We can get better at navigating consent in our sexual encounters by trying our best to ensure we are mindful of consent in every aspect of life, every day. Not only by making sure we feel sufficiently empowered to assert our own preferences but also by being mindful of the ways in which we participate in creating an atmosphere within which it may be difficult for someone else to decline what we ask of them, and actively working to instead create an environment where all parties can be honest without fearing their safety.

CONSENT 101: WHAT EVERYONE SHOULD KNOW

Consent needs to be willingly given. Pressurizing someone to do something you want to do when they don't want to do it is not consent.

Consent is specific, and seeking each other's consent needs to be an **ongoing process**. For example, agreeing to share a kiss or a cuddle does not automatically imply consent for intercourse. Consent to sex with a condom cannot be construed as consent to sex without a condom. We need to keep checking in with each other. Just because someone consents to one thing, don't assume you have their consent for another thing—ask. Also, consent once doesn't mean consent forever.

Consent is reversible. For example, you and your partner could have been excitedly planning to have sex, but then when you're actually in a room together, it might seem scary for one or both of you. It's okay for either of you to change your mind and say 'no'—consent can be reversed, and we've got to get better at respecting that.

Consent should be informed. Each person should be in a position to fully understand what they are consenting to. Alcohol and substance use, for example, can complicate consent. When under the influence of a substance, people are not in a position to give informed consent, so it is best not to initiate anything sexual.

Also, concealing information about your sexual health that may impact your partner's health and safety negates informed consent. For example, getting someone to agree to have unprotected sex by saying you've been tested for sexually transmitted infections when in fact you've never been tested, or you've been tested, and you know you have an infection, is a violation of consent.

If any party is either not in a position to comprehend what's being asked of them, or is being lied to or withheld relevant information from, when making a decision about whether to engage in something, it is not informed consent.

Power differentials such as major differences in age, authority or social and economic privilege are other important factors to consider. It can be especially hard to express not wanting to do something when the other person has much more power than you.

In a healthy relationship, one person doesn't have total control or get to automatically call all the shots—rather, both partners are equally able to voice their opinions, preferences and feelings. And both partners should have the right to withdraw consent at any point without having to fear for their safety, well-being or livelihood.

SAFER SEX: PROTECTION AND CONTRACEPTION

I think doing whatever you can to make sex safer is so damn sexy. Personally, I can't quite focus on my pleasure if I'm worried about the risks of pregnancy or sexually transmitted infections. It really is worth understanding what methods of protection and contraception are out there so that you can find the solution that is likely to work best for you and your partner.

Q What methods protect against both STIs and pregnancy?

Condoms—we will discuss both regular and internal condoms in a bit—are the only methods that can serve as protection against *both* pregnancy *and* STIs.

Contraceptives like birth control pills, the copper-T and the hormonal IUD—only protect against pregnancy. So if you and your partner haven't been tested for STIs, it's best to use a barrier method like a condom during intercourse, even if you're on some form of birth control.

And even during sexual activity that cannot result in a pregnancy—such as anal sex and oral sex—if both partners haven't been tested for STIs, using barrier methods like condoms and dental dams is very important, because STIs can be contracted from pretty much any activity that involves the sharing of bodily fluids.

Rather than scaring you though, this information is intended to equip you to make safer choices as far as possible—because, luckily, it's pretty easy to significantly reduce these risks.

Here's what's out there in terms of **barrier methods of protection**:

Regular Condoms

Worn on the penis. Can be used during:
- penetrative vaginal sex
- penetrative anal sex
- when a penis-owner receives oral sex. (Yes, it's advisable to use condoms even during blowjobs—that's why flavoured condoms exist!)

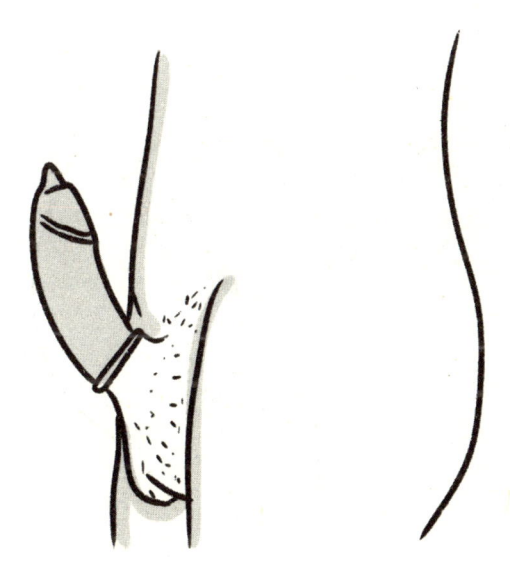

Internal Condoms

Worn inside the vagina or anus.

Can be used during:
- penetrative vaginal sex
- penetrative anal sex

Sometimes also called 'female condoms' because they are conceptualized to be worn internally rather than over a penis, they are a great option for people with vulvas seeking to take control of their own protection. They are typically wider than regular condoms, and have a larger outer rim that is meant to remain outside the vagina or anus, as well as a small inner ring, which helps in inserting the condom and keeping it in place.

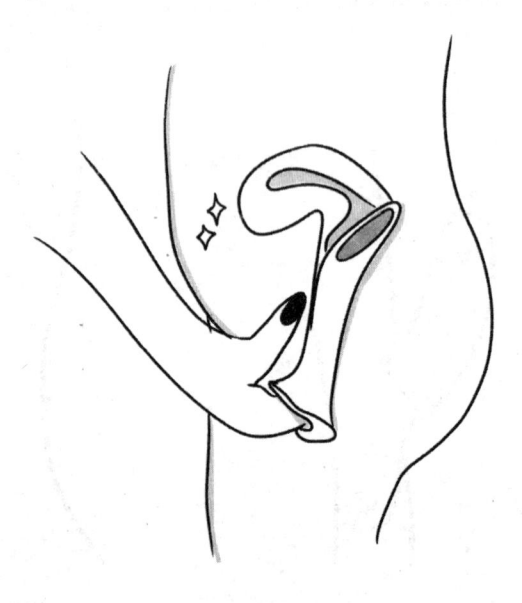

Use either a regular condom OR an internal condom, not both at the same time. Using both together does not double the protection—instead, it would make both condoms more likely to tear or get displaced.

Dental Dams

Essentially a small sheet of latex or polyurethane plastic, dental dams were actually used to isolate teeth from saliva during dental procedures—hence the name. But then people discovered they could also be used as barriers held in place to make **cunnilingus** (oral sex performed on a vulva usually with a particular focus on the clitoris) and **annilingus** (oral sex performed on an anus) safer. Since dental dams are kind of hard to find at stores, it's easy to make one yourself using a regular condom. With a clean pair of scissors, simply cut off the ring and the tip of a condom, and then cut along the length of the condom. You now have a rectangular piece of latex—your very own DIY dental dam!

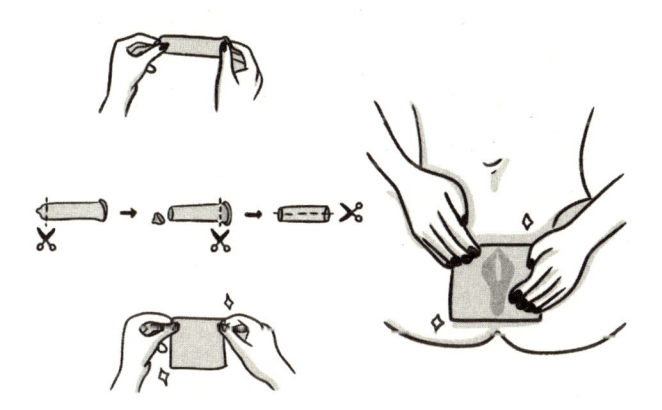

Condom FAQs

Q Ribbed, dotted, extra lubricated, climax delay, XL, flavoured? What type of condoms should one use?

Condoms are available in a bunch of different sizes and they generally come pre-lubricated. You can buy a few different brands and sizes to figure out what feels most comfortable and pleasurable for you.

Textured condoms—such as dotted or ribbed—are intended to enhance vaginal stimulation, and some people do enjoy how the added dimension of texture feels.

Be careful with **'climax delay' condoms**—they are often coated with lidocaine or other similar ingredients, which numb the penis to delay ejaculation—however, if used incorrectly they can numb your partner's vagina too.

Flavoured condoms are intended to be worn by a penis-owner receiving oral sex. They add an element of taste and flavour to make the idea of using a condom during a blowjob more fun. I would use non-flavoured condoms during vaginal intercourse as well as to make DIY dental dams, and use flavoured condoms only for BJs as the sugary coating on some flavoured condoms can disturb the vaginal ecosystem.

Q: Are some people allergic to condoms?

Most condoms are made of latex. A small percentage of people are allergic to latex.

However, if you do have a latex allergy, worry not—really great non-latex condoms made of materials like polyisoprene are also available. In fact, some people without latex allergies also prefer non-latex condom brands.

Q: How to put a condom on correctly? What if you put it on inside out?

When putting on a condom, make sure you don't accidentally put it on inside-out. The ring should be rolling up on the outside, rather than tucked in underneath. If you do accidentally have it positioned inside-out you will likely realize it as you try to roll it on—it's harder to roll down and it doesn't quite sit right. Throw it away and put on a new one. (In the off-chance that some precum or semen could have already gotten on the condom, you don't want to flip it around and use the same one.)

Q: Is it okay to switch between different sexual activities while using a condom?

Change condoms before switching from anal sex to vaginal sex—bacteria from the anus can cause infections if it enters the vagina. Also, as I mentioned, use regular, non-flavoured condoms for vaginal sex.

Q Is it okay to keep going after you ejaculate inside the condom?

Once the penis starts to become flaccid, the condom won't sit as taut, and semen can drip out. So it's best to carefully remove and dispose of the condom as soon after ejaculation as possible. Wash your penis and use a new condom if you resume sexual activity.

Q Any other condom best practices?

Store condoms away from direct sunlight and open condom sachets using your fingers, not scissors, so you don't accidentally damage the condom. And always check the expiry date.

My boyfriend always makes excuses not to wear a condom and often 'forgets' to bring them when we meet. I think 'pulling out' is too risky to rely on but he keeps trying to tell me that I'm unnecessarily paranoid. How can I make sure we have safe sex? – *Madhu*

Indeed, many men seem to like to 'forget' to bring condoms, and then suggest that the pull-out method is a foolproof option. It is not. It does not prevent STI transmission and technically, even precum can contain sperm. Plus, ejaculation isn't always easy to time precisely.

Still, among heterosexual couples, the decision to use protection often becomes one that rests almost entirely on the male partner's preference. Will he bring a condom? Even if he has one, will he use it?

Also, condom negotiation tends to be something that takes place in the heat of the moment—and if there aren't any condoms around, too often women don't feel empowered to object to unprotected sex.

Why not just keep your own box of condoms handy? Luckily, condoms are pretty widely accessible and relatively affordable—you can even order them online if you find it awkward buying them in person at the pharmacy or supermarket. Alternatively, you can look into wearing an internal condom. Internal condoms are also now more widely available in India than before, particularly online.

It's so important that women, too, are able to play an active role in navigating safer sex.

And men should stop thinking that they're doing women some great favour by wearing condoms. Men can get STIs too. To the dudes reading this—remember, you're also protecting *yourself.*

The fact that young adults, and particularly young women, are shamed for seeking out contraception blows my mind. It indicates that we're proactive and responsible about our health and safety. We should be applauded! It's unfortunate that instead, we have to fear being judged and condemned.

Buying condoms online is an option worth considering—more choice, less judgement. In an ideal world, all of us, regardless of our gender identity or sexual orientation, should be able to access contraception easily and safely.

As for a partner making excuses not to wear a condom—condoms are available in different sizes. So the 'I'm too big for condoms' argument is easily dismantled. Non-latex condoms are also available, so 'I'm allergic to latex' is another excuse that doesn't hold.

'It doesn't feel as good with a condom' is perhaps the most common excuse, a sentiment expressed not only by many men but, if we're honest, also by many people of all genders. However, I look at it this way: even the anxiety at the possibility, let alone the actuality, of contracting an infection or having an unwanted pregnancy, at least for me, definitely feels worse.

It's up to couples to decide for themselves what level of risk they are willing to take in their personal life, but I, for one, am very risk-averse in this department.

Also, if you put in a little bit of effort to figure out the condom size and material that is most comfortable for you and your partner, all kinds of sex can feel pretty damn great even with a condom on.

There are extra-thin condoms, extra-lubricated condoms—and some may even enhance sensations! Plus, even the actual act of putting on a condom can be rather fun and erotic if you choose to look at it that way. You could roll the condom on for your partner, for example, or try condoms in a textured material like ribbed or dotted, to add an element of novelty to the experience!

Contraception/Birth Control Methods Beyond Condoms

I'm keen to explore contraceptive options beyond condoms because I like how sex feels without condoms. I've also heard that, statistically, birth control pills and IUDs can reduce the risk of pregnancy even more than condoms. But I'm kind of scared of the idea of taking hormonal medication. What do you suggest? *Alana*

Many opposite-sex couples in long-term monogamous relationships consider switching from condoms to another method of contraception such as birth control pills or an IUD. Also, since with any reversible method of contraception, including condoms, there remains the small chance of human error or the incidence of contraceptive failure—if pregnancy is a concern—you might even consider another birth control method as an additional precaution along with condoms.

In either case, the first step is to see a doctor, so you can assess your health, medical history and your requirements, and they can explain what your options are.

Both partners should get tested for sexually transmitted infections. This is important because the other methods of contraception don't protect against STI transmission; they only protect against pregnancy. So, if STIs are a concern, condoms are non-negotiable.

Vasectomies and female sterilization are, of course, the most effective means of contraception; however, for people who might want to have kids at some point, or for those seeking a less invasive option, IUDs and implants are considered the most reliable long-acting reversible methods of birth control available. Oral contraceptive pills and contraceptive injections are also considered very effective when taken correctly.

Figuring out what contraception is best for you is determined by individual needs and preferences. Certain methods have contraindications based on health, personal medical history, lifestyle, family medical history, etc.—so you should consult a doctor to make your decision.

However, I do think we would all benefit from hearing about each other's experiences and normalizing such conversations, so I'm going to share my own experience navigating contraception for myself.

This is just me sharing my story, and should not be seen as medical advice.

I'm simply recounting my personal experience, and my own personal decision-making process. It might give you a sense of the sort of decision-making you, or you and your partner, can navigate together.

Heterosexual sex is an activity that brings with it the risk of unintended pregnancy. But birth control too comes with contraindications and side effects. Different people have different appetites for risk, and their own unique health and family circumstances, so people make a variety of different choices when it comes to using birth control.

Personally, the idea of kids is absolutely terrifying to me, so I've always been very proactive about using contraception, and eager to explore the methods available so as to determine the option that suits me best.

About ten years ago, when I first set out to figure out what birth control I could opt for in addition to condoms, the choices seemed pretty overwhelming, especially because they all came with side effects.

I have used the **copper-T**, the **progestin-only pill** and the **hormonal IUD**, so these are the methods I'll be talking about most.

The Copper-T

Initially, I felt sort of scared and reluctant to use a hormonal method—to many of us, the very idea of certain medications can seem scary, even though we might not actually know all that much about the medication in question. I told my gynaecologist that I wanted to explore a non-hormonal method first. She told me about the copper-T.

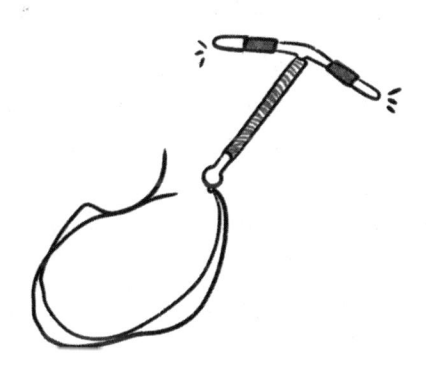

The copper IUD or intrauterine device is a T-shaped piece of plastic with copper coiled around it (hence popularly called the copper-T). It is manually inserted into your uterus by a doctor, and the insertion process takes just a few minutes. This can be painful in varying degrees for different people, but luckily for me, the process was totally bearable. How it works is that exposure to copper deactivates sperm, making it unable to fertilize an egg. Once inserted, the copper IUD can be used for up to over ten years.

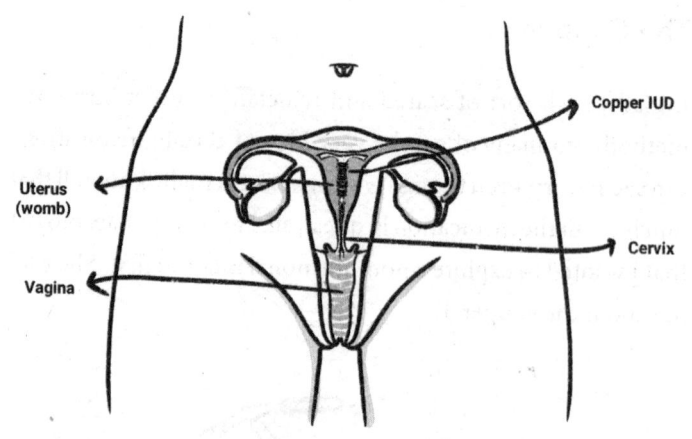

At the time, it seemed appealing to me because it was non-hormonal, low-cost, highly effective, and with the potential to be very long-lasting.

However, the copper IUD has some considerable side effects. For example, it tends to increase menstrual bleeding and menstrual cramps. Insertion can also be painful for some people.

While I had a hassle-free insertion process, over time, my much, much heavier periods and bad cramps really got to me. I felt weak and exhausted all the time. So I got it removed less than two years after I had it inserted, even though it can technically be used for over ten years.

I decided to try a hormonal method after I got the copper-T removed because I didn't really have much of a choice. As far as long-acting reversible contraceptives go, the copper IUD is basically the only non-hormonal method on offer.

My gynaecologist told me about birth control pills and about hormonal IUDs, but I decided I'd try the pill first. Having just had the copper IUD removed, I wanted to see how my body would react to hormonal pills before committing to a hormonal IUD.

Oral Contraceptive Pills

Birth control pills are typically formulated either with a combination of the hormones oestrogen and progestin, or progestin only.

The combination pill works primarily by preventing ovulation which is the release of an egg during the menstrual cycle. You can't get pregnant if you don't ovulate because there is no egg released to be fertilized.

Birth control pills can also work by thickening the mucus around the cervix, which makes it difficult for sperm to enter the uterus, and they can also sometimes affect the lining of the uterus, making it difficult for an egg to implant itself (attach to the wall of the uterus). All of this helps prevent pregnancy.

Factors like how old you are, if you smoke, and your medical history are very important in determining whether or not birth control pills are a viable option because there's a pretty long list of potential side effects, ranging from minor to severe.

Since I was a smoker, the oestrogen–progestin combined pill was not an option for me, as increased oestrogen levels from the combination pill together with smoking, can create a heightened risk of cardiovascular health problems. So instead, I was prescribed the progestin-only pill, and I took it for over a year.

Birth control pills are taken orally, so there is no potentially painful insertion process, unlike with the IUD. However, this 'pro', at least in my books, is also in some ways a 'con'. You have to remember to take the pill every day, ideally at the same time, for it to work.

Having to think about birth control every day, with an alarm and all of that, just felt annoying and stressful for me, personally.

Some birth control pills are known to help with the symptoms of PCOS as well as with managing severe acne, but others can exacerbate menstrual irregularities and symptoms.

When I was on the progestin-only pill, I experienced increased mood swings, headaches, bloating and acne.

Overall, for me, it just wasn't quite as hassle free as I was hoping it would be.

Around the same time that I decided I wanted to switch from the pill to something else, I learned that a close friend of mine had a hormonal IUD and had been on it for years.

She said she had had a really positive experience. I decided to explore that option with my gynac, who concurred that it is widely thought of as among the best contraceptive methods available.

Hormonal IUDs

Hormonal IUDs look very similar to copper IUDs in shape, and have the same sort of insertion process, but the difference is that, instead of copper, they use a hormone to prevent pregnancy.

Hormonal IUDs can last for three to seven years once inserted. They work by releasing a small amount of hormone called levonorgestrel (a type of progestin) directly into the uterus. (The daily amount of hormone released is smaller than the amount you'd consume orally with a birth control pill as it is released locally.)

The hormone released by hormonal IUDs works either by thickening the mucus on your cervix to stop sperm from reaching an egg and/or by suppressing ovulation.

Unlike the copper IUD, hormonal IUDs typically decrease the severity of periods, and some people even stop getting their period altogether. For some, this might sound disconcerting, but to me, having dealt with the excessively heavy periods that came with the copper IUD, this seemed like a major advantage.

Hormonal IUDs are considerably more expensive than copper IUDs and are effective for a slightly shorter number of years, but it is a one-time cost and, unlike with the copper-T, I have not yet had to remove it, and it's been over four years since the insertion. So far, overall, it's the method I've been happiest with. (I have the Mirena IUD.)

I got over my somewhat unexamined initial fear of 'hormonal' birth control the hard way—I tried the non-hormonal methods first and found that, at least for me, they weren't ideal.

For me, the insertion process was slightly painful, but not unbearable. It took only a couple of minutes, and I was able to go back to work after my appointment.

Over the first couple of months after getting my hormonal IUD I did experience some irregular bleeding—but after that, I have not really had to think about it much. And my period has become so light that I rarely really need more than a pantyliner as far as my use of period products goes. For me, this has been a huge plus.

IUDs are reversible—you can have your gynaecologist remove it at any point, and your fertility goes back to normal.

Given my personal experience, it surprises me that hormonal IUDs aren't more popular—somehow, I also discovered it only after first trying other methods.

There's definitely a lack of information, a stigma around products that require vaginal insertion and an exaggerated perception that IUDs are dangerous, partly because there was a faulty American model called the Dalkon Shield launched in the seventies that was terrible.

But the current hormonal IUDs are considered among the most effective and hassle-free, long-acting, reversible methods of birth control and so it's an option worth researching and discussing with your doctor if you're navigating contraception beyond condoms.

There are additional contraceptive options such as patches, injections, implants and more—but I haven't used any of these myself. They all have their own pros and cons, and it's worth doing your research and talking to your gynaecologist to explore what might work best for you.

All of this said, I do think choosing contraception can feel like a less-than-ideal experience—it's like you're having to figure out which option sucks the least. There isn't yet a perfect, 100 per cent effective, zero side effects option. And you have to weigh the severity of those potential side effects against the possibility of an unintended pregnancy, and make a decision.

It's terribly unfair that the physical, emotional and financial costs of birth control are something women and people with uteruses have to deal with so disproportionately—as also with the consequences of an accidental pregnancy.

For an activity that men and people with penises equally participate in, it is unfair that the potential consequences, both of contraceptive medication as well as the absence of it, tend to land squarely on the lives and bodies of women and people with vulvas.

We should all advocate for new and safer contraceptive methods, and for dependable, long-acting, reversible birth control for people with penises too.

We need better. We deserve better. And we should demand more, so that future generations have better options. And in order for that to happen, we need to at the very least be having this conversation.

Q What's the difference between birth control pills, emergency contraception/ 'i-pill' and abortion pills?

Because we rarely talk about this stuff openly, people are often quite confused about these medications—but in the interest of better sexual health and safety, this really deserves to be common knowledge.

Each of these medications is different and serves its own specific purpose.

You can think of birth control pills as prevention. They are a hormonal medication taken daily as a primary form of contraception to prevent your body from being capable of getting pregnant even when sexually active.

In order to work effectively to prevent pregnancy, this medication needs to start being taken at least a week *before* you engage in unprotected sexual activity, and it is to be taken daily—ideally at the same time each day—on an ongoing basis.

You have to take it every day whether or not you are having sex that day, in order for it to offer protection whenever you do have sex.

When taken correctly, they are highly effective at preventing pregnancy. But if you stop taking them, you can get pregnant, and you also run the risk of pregnancy if you take them irregularly.

If you are already pregnant, birth control pills cannot be used to terminate a pregnancy.

You can think of emergency contraception as interception. In India, it is commonly called the 'i-pill' as that's the name of one of the most widely available brands of this medication.

It is intended for use only in 'emergencies'—typically when a primary form of contraception such as condoms or birth control pills was not used correctly or not used at all. And therefore, it is often colloquially called the 'morning-after pill' or, as in the US, 'Plan B'.

In order to be most likely to work, an emergency contraceptive pill needs to be taken **as soon after sex as possible**—before a pregnancy has taken place. It can be taken up to five days after intercourse, but the sooner it is taken, the more likely it is to be effective.

The emergency contraceptive pill or 'i-pill' is not the same as the abortion pill and is not effective beyond 120 hours after intercourse.

Relying on using emergency contraception *after* having sex is significantly less effective at preventing pregnancy than having a **primary form of contraception** in place *before* having sex—such as condoms, birth control pills or IUDs. It therefore should not be used as your go-to method of contraception, but rather only relied upon in emergencies, because far more effective methods of primary contraception exist.

You can think of abortion pills or medical abortion as termination—this medication, typically a combination of pills containing mifepristone and misoprostol, is taken only **after a pregnancy has already occurred**, for early-stage abortions.

A medical abortion with pills works by blocking the hormones necessary for maintaining a pregnancy and stimulating the uterus to expel the pregnancy.

Medical abortions are considered very safe and are most often prescribed for abortions taking place within the first trimester of a pregnancy. (For later-stage abortions, surgical abortion may be prescribed.)

Abortion pills are not the same thing as birth control or emergency contraception.

UNDERSTANDING ABORTION IN INDIA

A few weeks ago, my partner and I had sex and the condom broke. I should have gotten my period by now, but it hasn't come, so we got a pregnancy test, and it turns out I'm pregnant. I'm a nervous wreck right now. I know I am in no position to become a parent. I want an abortion. I never thought I would ever be in this situation so I literally have

no idea how to go about it. I feel so alone. Please help!
– Maya

An accidental pregnancy can happen to anyone. And anyone in such a situation deserves support, not stigma.

In the absence of comprehensive sex education, information about safer sex practices, and still-looming barriers to accessing contraception—social taboos, affordability, availability—as well as the fact that contraceptive failure can and does occur, and that sexual decision-making is not as simple and straightforward a process as we'd like to imagine, unplanned pregnancy is, in fact, extremely common.

Even though millions of abortions take place around the world and in India each year, it remains something that's shrouded in shame and misinformation. And that needs to change.

I had the privilege of talking to Dr Nozer Sheriar, one of India's most respected gynaecologists and a globally celebrated champion of sexual and reproductive health and rights, to understand the legal and medical frameworks around abortion in India. Here are the answers to several important questions about what an abortion in India entails:

Q Is abortion legal in India?

Abortion is legal in India. Under the Medical Termination of Pregnancy Act or MTP Act of 1971, abortion is legal in India up to twenty weeks into a pregnancy. This Act was amended in

2021 to increase the upper gestation limit for certain 'vulnerable categories' including survivors of rape, minors and people with disabilities, to up to twenty-four weeks into a pregnancy.

The law states that an abortion can be obtained in **any** of the following scenarios:

1. the pregnancy poses a threat to the life of the pregnant person
2. the pregnancy poses a threat to the physical or mental health of the pregnant person
3. if there are foetal abnormalities present
4. in cases of contraceptive failure

So, in theory, anyone seeking to terminate their pregnancy should be able to legally obtain a safe abortion in India.

However, it remains at the behest of doctors, rather than solely at the request of the pregnant person.

Up to twenty weeks into a pregnancy, the law requires a person to have the authorization of one medical provider in order to obtain an abortion. Between twenty and twenty-four weeks, however, the authorization of two medical providers is required.

If the pregnancy poses a risk to the pregnant person's life, the upper gestation limit does not apply, and an abortion can be done at any stage in the pregnancy.

In cases where there are foetal abnormalities, the upper gestation limit also does not apply; however, the authorization of a medical board is required.

Q Can you get an abortion if you are not married?

You do not have to be married to obtain an abortion in India. Moreover, according to the law, a person who is eighteen years or older and sound of mind does not need the permission of their parents, spouse or anyone other than their doctors to get an abortion. They can also be assured that their identity will be kept confidential.

Q Can you get an abortion if you are under the age of eighteen?

This is a more complicated question. In India, the legal 'age of consent' for sex is 18— which effectively criminalizes all sex by people under the age of eighteen, even if it is consensual.

The Protection of Children from Sexual Offences (POCSO) Act, which is intended to protect children and young people from sexual abuse, is an important and valuable Act. However, it does not currently differentiate between consensual sexual activity between teenagers similar in age, and non-consensual sexual activity, or sexual activity between an adult and a minor. So, even though licensed medical practitioners can perform an abortion for a person under eighteen years of age, they are legally required to file a police report even if the sex was consensual.

We need to advocate for a solution to this so that young people who may need it can access safe abortion without involving the police—because, let's be honest, this law isn't going to make teenagers stop having sex. It's only going to force them to opt for unsafe abortions outside of the healthcare system.

Q How safe is abortion?

When performed correctly, abortions, particularly early-stage abortions, are very, very safe. In fact, abortion is considered among the safest procedures in obstetric practice. To give you a sense of how safe it is—statistically, it is a safer procedure than delivering a child. It's also worth keeping in mind that, generally, safe abortions do not impact a person's long-term fertility.

Q What sort of procedures does a safe abortion entail?

In the early stages of a pregnancy, medical abortions or abortion pills can simply be taken orally. Tablets of mifepristone and misoprostol are usually taken in two phases, and these medications help terminate and expel the pregnancy.

The other option in the first trimester is suction aspiration, which is a simple surgical procedure involving either a manual aspirator or an electrically operated device which uses gentle suction to remove the pregnancy.

For later-stage abortions, slightly more elaborate surgical procedures are required, but around 90 per cent of abortions take place in the first trimester.

Q Are abortions painful?

This depends on what procedure is opted for, and what stage of the pregnancy the person is in.

Medical abortions with pills, which can be done in the early stages of a pregnancy, can be painful, as when the uterus expels the pregnancy, one might experience pain similar to severe period cramps. But doctors also provide pain-management and pain-relief solutions.

Surgical abortion procedures, typically done if the pregnancy is in a later stage, are done with anaesthesia.

Q How common is abortion?

Abortion is much more common than you probably think. It is estimated by the Guttmacher Institute that has the most credible studies on the subject, that at least 56 million abortions take place across the world annually,[6] and at least 15.6 million abortions take place in India each year.[7]

---

6 https://www.guttmacher.org/report/abortion-unintended-pregnancy-six-states-india

7 https://www.guttmacher.org/news-release/2017/national-estimate-abortion-india-released

Simply going by the statistics, abortion is so common, in fact, that it is highly likely that someone both in your family and in my family has already had an abortion. So if you are someone going through this, know that you are not alone.

Q Why is it important that we support the right to choose?

Even today, abortion in India is not considered a human right and people continue to face challenges while accessing safe abortion services.

According to the MTP Act, abortion needs the opinion and approval of a medical practitioner. A person cannot get an abortion solely on their request. This is reflective of the prevalent socio-cultural and legal perception that a woman cannot and should not control her own reproductive choices.

These attitudes sometimes extend even to providers, who often ask for spousal or family consent before providing an abortion though it is not a legal requirement. Biases such as these further prevent people from accessing safe abortion.

Denying people access to safe abortion is not going to magically stop unwanted pregnancies. It only stands to jeopardize the health and lives of millions of people around the world by forcing them to seek potentially dangerous solutions outside of the healthcare system. *Unsafe abortion is still among the leading causes of maternal death in our country.*

On a fundamental level, every human being deserves sexual and bodily autonomy—we deserve the right to make our own choices about our own bodies. If we have any value for our own agency and bodily autonomy, access to safe abortion is a right we should all be advocating for globally.

EMOTIONAL SAFETY

When we talk about safer sex the focus is usually only on physical safety: managing the risks of infection and pregnancy. I think it's important that we also begin considering our emotional well-being. How can we ensure that our sexual experiences feel fulfilling and safe emotionally too? How can we make our sexual experiences feel kinder and more respectful, memorable and fun?

Understanding 'Aftercare'

Whether it's a casual encounter, sex with your long-term partner, or anything in-between, how partners respond after sex can affect whether you feel safe and comfortable, confused, or upset.

This is why the concept of sexual 'aftercare' is helpful. Discussing with one another how you each like to interact post sex is a valuable conversation to have. Whether you like cuddling or you need some space, whether you like talking, or you'd rather be quiet—these are things you can discuss so that you're each able to understand one another's needs and behaviours better.

Rolling over and avoiding your partner or leaving right after sex, for example, can sometimes make the other person feel used or undervalued. On the other hand, long-drawn snuggles might be too much intimacy for some people, especially if you're just getting to know each other; others might love it. So it's worth talking about this stuff.

Even simply getting a cup of tea together after sex can make such a world of difference in terms of whether a sexual experience feels positive and memorable or confusing and upsetting.

Feelings are not embarrassing!

For young people navigating current-day dating culture, it can often seem like 'catching feels' is something to be avoided at all costs. Many of us are terrified of seeming 'needy' or 'attached', or exposing our vulnerabilities, particularly during a sexual or romantic interaction, and especially if the encounter is understood to be 'casual'.

Perhaps some of this trepidation around feelings comes from wanting to avoid getting hurt—but we deny ourselves genuine human connection when we treat each other like disposable objects instead of treating each other with respect and empathy.

Whether it's a casual hook-up, a relationship of many years, or anything in between, we'd all have much more fulfilling experiences if we get better at expressing and processing our emotions instead of hiding from them.

Feelings are not embarrassing. They're what make us human. Our most fulfilling interactions tend to be those where we feel comfortable being our true selves.

We don't owe it to one another to always reciprocate a feeling, but we can certainly at least remember our shared humanity.

Q Why do people sometimes cry after sex?

Crying is a natural bodily response to big feelings, and sex can be an emotionally intense experience.

Sometimes tearing up could simply be a response to the joyful overwhelm of an extremely pleasurable encounter and a sense of deep connection and intimacy. Sometimes it may be the result of difficult feelings that arise from past sexual trauma or feelings of discomfort or shame around sex. For some people it may be a part of trying to process an aspect of the relationship. Whatever the reason, it's okay to cry.

It would be wonderful if we could all be compassionate with ourselves and each other when sex brings up emotion.

Pleasure

Everyone Deserves It!

I once had the privilege of listening to a talk by the magnificent contemporary philosopher, Zhenevere Sophia Dao, about sexuality, identity and pleasure—and she made this fascinating point: If you were to say that you work for twenty hours a day, you'd be applauded; if you were to say you go to the gym for three hours a day, you'd be applauded. But if you were to say you make sure to allocate even just one hour every day for self-pleasure, or to better understand and celebrate your sexuality, you'd likely be ridiculed or dismissed. You'd likely be shamed and made to wonder whether something is wrong with you. You'd perhaps be made to feel like a 'freak', or guilty for 'wasting' your time.

Think about how messed up that is. We are encouraged to see our bodies as something to make as 'functional' and as 'productive' as possible. So work is great, gym is great. But pleasure? Pleasure is 'shameful'; 'wasteful'; 'unproductive'.

Why are we made to think of honouring our own pleasure as something embarrassing, dirty, lesser-than, freakish, a waste of time—as opposed to something joyful, something important, something sublime?

How can we change that narrative? How can we begin to see sexual pleasure, including self-pleasure, as something important and valuable?

Also, too often, sex education is focused on abstinence and inculcating fear—fear of pregnancy, fear of disease, fear of violence. Even when well-intentioned, this approach tends to only consider the question of how to prevent negative sexual experiences. Not how to ensure joyful ones.

While of course these are important concerns that we absolutely ought to address—and I believe I have addressed them in this book—in addition to doing what we can to prevent the negatives, I also want to talk about what we can do to enable the most gloriously pleasurable experiences.

Because, if we're honest, pleasure is one of the foremost motivations for why people have sex. Of all the people engaging in sexual activity right now across the world, only a fraction are doing so with the express intention of having a baby. Most are likely doing it because it makes them feel good.

So when we talk in educational contexts about sex, why do we never talk about pleasure? If pleasure does get a mention, why is it typically only cishet men's pleasure? How can we not only make pleasure part of the conversation but also expand our understanding of pleasure so that it becomes more inclusive and gender equal?

How can we ensure that all our sexual experiences are gloriously pleasurable?

These are some of the questions this next section will seek to unravel.

SELF-PLEASURE

Cultivating a Self-pleasure Practice as a Gateway to Sexual Self-knowledge

Up until my late twenties, my own pleasure seemed incredibly mysterious to me.

During intercourse, it took so much effort to even attempt to reach orgasm; it was so hit or miss, that most of the time, I'd end up just faking it.

Women's pleasure has long been characterized in sex and relationship advice columns as 'difficult', 'complicated', 'unlikely to happen every time', 'too much to ask for'. So I thought that just *is how it is*.

In the unlikely event that a partner was both generous and skilled at cunnilingus, I found that I was far more likely to have a good time. However, even then, I was often too busy worrying about how I look and taste and smell to fully enjoy myself.

Then, one evening, I was chatting at a party with a friend who is bisexual. She had been in a relationship with a woman for the last couple of years; they'd broken up a few months ago and she had recently developed a crush on a man, but after getting physical with him she was terribly disappointed.

'How do you straight girls manage?' she asked incredulously. 'He had no clue what he was doing! I'd forgotten how much straight guys need to be schooled! I don't think I'm going to bother having casual sex with a dude again after this—my vibrator is *so fantastic*, and I don't even have to shave my legs!'

I had never owned a vibrator and I had no idea what I was missing. But if the look in my friend's eyes when she talked about hers was anything to go by, clearly I was missing a lot. I asked her to tell me all about it.

'Sex with a guy who has no idea how your body works, when you have a vibrator at home, is quite literally like choosing to take the bus when you own a Ferrari,' she laughed.

'Even the most highly skilled lover can't compete with the speed and consistency. It's just a massive technological upgrade from anything a human can do. I know it's a machine, and of course, it can't replace the amazing sense of care and connection that comes with a great relationship, but it sure beats bad sex with some random dude who can't be bothered to figure out what makes you feel good. My vibrator has taught me *so much* about the extent of the pleasure my body is capable of!'

All through my teenage years, I had never masturbated—I'd internalized all the ridiculous messaging about it being a silly, shameful thing to do, and an inferior substitute to 'real' sex.

And as I entered adulthood and had my first sexual relationships, I thought since I was having partnered sex, surely I had no need for masturbation.

It was only just beginning to dawn on me how mistaken I'd been.

Why was I ashamed to explore my pleasure on my own? And did I even know enough about my own pleasure to be able to make it a genuine priority during partnered sex?

As soon as I got home that night, I scoured the internet for how to buy sex toys in India and promptly ordered the best vibrator I could afford. (Since this was several years ago, there was significantly less choice than there is now.)

Still, I found something rather life-altering.

It was a dual-action 'rabbit'-style vibrator—one that can provide both intense clitoral and rumbly vaginal stimulation simultaneously. And yes, I am pleased to report that it does feel every bit as toe-curlingly satisfying as it sounds.

Since we're on the topic of toys—a quick aside here before I continue on the subject of my own sexual self-discovery—the 'rabbit' design has actually been around for decades. Having become quite the toy aficionado at this point, when I look at my old rabbit vibe now, I've got to admit it's rather crude-looking in comparison to the sleek and abstract aesthetics that more contemporary sex tech has adopted—so you might want to try a newer design if you're inspired to buy your first vibrator. That said, the rabbit certainly still manages to get the job done.

The first time I used it, I was so struck by what I experienced that I thought if I could make one wish right now, I would wish that it rained vibrators—so everyone on the planet with a vulva could have one. I couldn't believe that up until this point I didn't even know how much pleasure my body was capable of.

Vibrators are *incredibly* effective at stimulating the vulva, particularly the external clitoris. For me, having an orgasm during partnered penetrative sex typically required a meticulous combination of oral sex and fingering beforehand and just the right angle thereafter, and so, reaching orgasm would take at least thirty minutes or more overall—if it even happened at all.

With a vibrator, you're likely to be able to orgasm in a matter of minutes if you want to. Every. Time.

Also, if like me, you too proceeded into your first sexual relationships without having ever really masturbated, here's the other discovery I made when I finally got started: There's just something about doing an activity alone rather than in the presence of another person.

Consider even an activity as banal and everyday as eating. Don't you sometimes eat a bit differently in front of people than you might when you're on your own? And sometimes, don't you just want to eat chocolate ice cream straight from the tub, as much of it and as messily as you want, without anyone watching you?

It takes a spectacularly high level of self-confidence and self-awareness to do any task in front of another person exactly the way you would when you're on your own. I realized that this can be particularly true of sex, especially with a new partner.

Cultivating a self-pleasure practice, especially for vulva-owners (most penis-owners cultivate one anyway), can be a wonderful entryway into discovering your own body and pleasure minus the pressure of any expectations or insecurities that often become magnified when you're with a partner you want to please and impress.

After years of believing my pleasure was inscrutable and elusive, I discovered that it is actually not 'difficult' at all. I simply hadn't known enough about how my body works, and the cultural messaging around how women should experience sex had been inaccurate and misleading.

I learned more about my pleasure and my body over the year that I bought my vibrator than I had over all previous years of being sexually active combined. It has literally been a revelation.

I also got so much better at being able to articulate my preferences during partnered sex. Equipped with the newfound knowledge about how my body works in relation to pleasure, I was able to communicate with my partner much more confidently and effectively.

Too often as women we're made to feel like we ought to downplay or hide our sexuality and desires—even when we do know what makes us feel good, we may hesitate to instruct our partners or ask for what we want.

Men, on the other hand, are encouraged to present themselves as sexually assertive and knowledgeable, even if they don't actually know what they're doing.

By exploring my pleasure solo, I was able to better understand the most intimate parts of my body and, as a result, I became much more expressive in my romantic life.

After all, if we don't discover and share what works for us, how can we expect our partners to know?

In fact, since I'm really baring my soul (or is it my vagina?) here, I might as well tell you that cultivating a self-pleasure practice for the first time in my life in my late twenties had such a profound impact on me that it really galvanized the creation of my digital platforms focused on pleasure-centric sex education five years ago.

I had long wanted to create free and accessible sex ed resources, but it was this experience of self-discovery and pleasure that was the tipping point. It was like, Oh. My. Gosh. How did I not know this—how did I not know that I could feel *this much* pleasure? There must be so many people out there who still don't know. Time to shout it from the rooftops!

But let me also say this: while it's certainly worth acquainting yourself with your own genitals, there's also lots more to sexual pleasure than just the penis and vulva. Many people of all genders experience intense pleasure from things like kissing, nipple stimulation, stimulation of the ears, neck or back, stimulation of the core muscles, stimulation of the feet and, believe it or not, even via meditation.

Slowly, thoughtfully figuring out your arousal can be a hugely fulfilling experience.

Remember, your body is a treasure trove of pleasure. Go forth and explore!

Q I've never masturbated. How do I go about it? How do most people masturbate?

I get this question pretty frequently, mainly from women. Most people masturbate using their hands or toys to touch their genitals in ways that feel pleasurable to them. People with penises typically stroke their penis, and people with vulvas typically rub their clitoris and/or finger their vagina, or use a vibrator to stimulate these parts.

That said, some people may prefer masturbating without using their hands or toys. A lot of women and vulva-owners discover the pleasure of masturbation, sometimes unknowingly, by simply squeezing or clenching their thighs together while sitting or lying down. For some, this can create pleasurable pressure on the clitoris and vagina. Some people may even enjoy simply rubbing up against their bed or a pillow.

Many people enjoy watching porn or reading erotica to feel aroused in the lead-up to or during masturbation, but personally, I prefer using my imagination.

If you have a vulva and you've never masturbated but are keen to try it, I highly recommend taking a proper look at your vulva using a hand mirror and familiarizing yourself with the parts. Identify your clitoris, try rubbing or tickling it. Gently explore how it feels to have a finger inside your vagina if you like. (Make sure your hands are clean and that your nails aren't sharp.) The section in this book on the anatomy of the vulva may be helpful to refer to when trying to figure out which bit does what (see page 18).

You could get yourself a vibrator and see if you like how the sensation of vibration feels on your external clitoris (it tends to feel pretty magical!). If it's a toy that's also suitable for internal use, then see how it feels when inserted. (Make sure your toy is made of a body-safe material, and make sure to clean your toy before and after use.)

Many people with vulvas experience their first orgasm when using a vibrating toy on their external clitoris. As I've said, they're exceptionally effective at clitoral stimulation. Dual-action toys that provide external clitoral and internal vaginal stimulation simultaneously can also feel fantastic.

Whether you have a vulva or a penis, lube can be a great addition to your self-pleasure routine. It makes things feel delightfully smooth and slidey-glidey.

More on both toys and lube shortly. (If it isn't clear already, I'm a huge fan!)

And while, of course, the genitals have a lot of pleasure to offer, don't ignore the rest of your body—take the time to explore all the places where touch feels good! You'll be pleasantly surprised at how soothing it can feel even to lovingly massage your own arms, legs or breasts.

If you're feeling fancy, turn the lights down low, light a scented candle, play some sexy music. It can be lovely to set the mood even for some solo pleasure—you don't have to have a date to put in the effort to make things feel special. You are reason enough!

Q Is it okay to masturbate even if you're in a relationship?

We're taught to see masturbation as some sort of inferior substitute for partnered sex. Some people even mistakenly think that masturbating when you're in a relationship amounts to cheating.

Masturbation isn't necessarily a substitute for sex; it is its own activity. And for people in relationships, it doesn't have to be one or the other. It's okay to masturbate regardless of whether or not you're in a relationship. Surely each of us deserves the irrevocable right and freedom to soothe, explore and pleasure our own bodies in our own private space, without harming anyone, whether or not we're in a relationship.

In fact, if my DMs are anything to go by, many women report that masturbating translated into more exciting partnered sex too because it made them more aware of how their own bodies work in relation to pleasure, and more confident discussing their preferences in bed. This was certainly my experience as well.

Additionally, while most people see masturbation as a necessarily solitary activity, it's worth considering the fact that masturbation can also be a partnered activity. **Mutual masturbation** can be a rather enjoyable experience if you and your partner are open to trying it together.

Q What is mutual masturbation?

Mutual masturbation can refer to either of two things:

1. When you and your partner stimulate each other's body or genitals with your hands or with toys.

OR

2. When you and your partner each stimulate your own body or genitals with your hands or with toys in each other's presence.

This second version of mutual masturbation—where partners basically masturbate in front of each other—can be a great way to better understand each other's pleasure. It allows each partner to show the other exactly how they like to be touched. It's also a very safe form of experiencing sexual pleasure—there's no danger of accidental pregnancy or STIs.

Masturbating in front of your partner can seem intimidating or 'weird' at first because, as we've discussed, masturbation is usually seen as something very private, that you do alone. But once you wrap your head around the idea of mutual masturbation, it can actually feel extremely intimate for the exact same reason. It establishes that you and your partner are very comfortable with each other, and it can be a fantastic way to learn about each other's bodies and pleasure.

Here are some delightful messages I've received from people on the unique potential that mutual masturbation provides for the navigation of pleasure:

Since I'm in a long-distance relationship, my boyfriend and I have had to rely almost entirely on mutual masturbation—although virtually—for like two years now.

I've got to say, mutual masturbation even on a video call with your partner can be pretty hot, and I'm sure it's thanks to these sessions that his technique has gotten so good at making me orgasm when we're together in person. – *Lily*

I'm a sexual-assault survivor and, over the pandemic, we have done a lot of mutual masturbation via phone sex and it's created a safe space for us to a) explore fantasies

together and b) for me to push boundaries of what I'm okay with (and not!) because it's reduced the risk of me freezing or my body shutting down. I've found myself being honest and sexy and open about what I enjoy and I have, finally, after a long time, asserted my right to sexual pleasure. I've also spent some wonderful hours exploring what makes him happy. It's wonderful and I highly recommend it to couples, especially where one or both partners carry trauma with them. It creates an open, conducive space for intimacy and vulnerability. – *Sanjana*

Mutual masturbation is great—it's pretty much the only way I know I'll have an orgasm during sex. I like to think of not just traditional 'foreplay' as foreplay, but even penetration as my foreplay—and then once he finishes, I LOVE using a vibrator to bring myself to orgasm while my partner watches! – *Shimouli*

ORGASMS

Q What is an orgasm exactly, and how do I know if I've had one?

I get this question *a lot*, particularly from people with vulvas. Because of how ignored our pleasure has been and tends to continue to be within heteronormative sexual scripts, many of us have never had an orgasm, or are left wondering if we've ever had one, well into our adult lives. So, first of all, if you have this question, know that you are not alone.

An orgasm is a sort of peak state of sexual arousal and pleasure that can be experienced both via solo and partnered sexual activity. Your muscles may contract, and your heart rate and breathing are likely to intensify as your body and mind build up your sexual arousal to a feeling of climax, followed by a feeling of release.

For people with penises, orgasm is typically accompanied by the literal release of ejaculate and sometimes a release of fluid may accompany orgasm even for people with vulvas. (More on squirting and female ejaculate on page 191.)

During pleasurable sex and orgasm, 'feel-good hormones' like oxytocin, dopamine and endorphins are typically released in the brain, and so people often feel happy, light-headed, emotional or sleepy in the aftermath of climax.

Still, these explanations have their limitations, because an orgasm can be one of those sensorially and emotionally explosive things that's just rather hard to describe precisely in words without ending up limiting rather than revealing its definition.

I love exploring the origins and meanings of words, so bear with me while I indulge my inner linguistics nerd here for a minute.

While the word *orgasm* derives etymologically from the Greek word *orgasmos* which means swelling and excitement, in a paper titled 'Behold, I Am Coming Soon!: A Study on the Conceptualization of Sexual Orgasm in 27 Languages',[8] researchers Anita Yen Chiang and Wen-yu Chiang note that 'orgasm' across cultures has been conceptualized in a variety of related but subtly different ways: 'as a physiological response, a psychological state, and as an ideal goal'.

From Farsi to Finnish, from Bengali to Tagalog, they list the key metaphors around how orgasm has been conceptualized linguistically: orgasm as a peak or summit; orgasm as fire; orgasm as arriving at a destination; orgasm as an end or a departure; orgasm as a release of force or substance; and orgasm as a feeling of intense satisfaction.

Indeed, even in Hindi, the phrase *charam sukh prapti* suggests a sort of apex of pleasure and satisfaction.

If you've had an orgasm, you can probably relate to these framings of the body tingling with fiery pleasure, bringing forth a physical and often even emotional catharsis.

The French phrase for orgasm—*la petite mort*—means 'the little death'. A fascinating phrase, it points to long-standing philosophical associations of the erotic with the tragic, and of sex as something both *worldly, bodily, base* as well as *otherworldly, exquisite, transcendental*.

Whether solo or partnered, sexual activity is often most pleasurable, and orgasms most likely to occur, when there's

---

[8] 'Behold, I Am Coming Soon! A Study on the Conceptualization of Sexual Orgasm in 27 Languages', Anita Yen Chiang and Wen-yu Chiang, 31:3, 131-147, DOI. 10.1080/10926488.2016.1187043

an adequate build-up of pleasure, a gradual escalation. This process of 'getting warmed up' is often called 'foreplay'.

FOREPLAY

Q What is 'foreplay'?

Foreplay traditionally refers to sexual acts other than penetration—kissing, cuddling, breast play, fingering, oral sex, etc.—suggesting that these are acts that should take place in the lead-up to penetration. And while it does indeed help tremendously to ensure you and your partner feel sufficiently aroused before attempting penetrative sex of any kind, the word 'foreplay' can make it sound like these acts are only some sort of optional precursors to the 'main event' when, in fact, these acts themselves can be incredibly pleasurable, sometimes even more pleasurable than penetration, and can very well be the main event too!

I also want to share two powerful insights around foreplay that have stayed with me ever since I first read them: one from Dr Laurie Mintz, whom I've quoted before, and the other from award-winning relationship expert and couples therapist, Esther Perel.

Here's Dr Laurie on how the very language we use to describe sexual activity is, by default, focused around male pleasure—and hence the limitations of the word 'foreplay':

'If women's sexual satisfaction were the defining criteria [in the language we use around sex], intercourse wouldn't be the "main event". Foreplay would be. The clitoral caressing that occurs before intercourse would be called sex and intercourse would be called post-play.'

And here's Esther Perel[9] on rethinking foreplay to include much more than just the physical sexual acts that occur before penetration:

> Foreplay is so much more than just the physical suggestion that kick-starts a sexual encounter. Foreplay is the energy that runs through an entire relationship. It begins at the end of the previous orgasm and it lives as an ever-present suggestion that a small look, touch, text or banter might lead to a little more. Foreplay is a mood we live in, a way we look at ourselves, how we feel about ourselves in the presence of a lover—or even in the presence of just our own reflection. At its core, great foreplay is made of the same things that make play, in general, so fun—exploring, creating, bonding, and trying new things.

KISSING

How to Be a 'Good Kisser'

Kissing is one of my most favourite acts of intimacy. Long, passionate kisses while holding each other's faces, or caressing

---

9   You can read this and more from Esther Perel on foreplay here: https://www.estherperel.com/blog/rethinking-foreplay

each other's hair—just the thought can make me swoon. Deep kissing in the lead-up to, and during intercourse can greatly intensify pleasure.

Being a 'good kisser' requires communication. Do you like soft, delicate kisses, or do you like getting your tongues in a frenzy together? Do you like sucking on each other's lips, or do you only like lips gently touching each other? Do you like your partner's hands around your waist, or supporting your head, or all over your body while they kiss you? Tell each other!

If you're new to kissing and aren't yet sure how to go about it, starting slow and soft is always a good idea. You can together work your way up to a more intense proximity and tempo if you're both into it!

Indeed, at the start of a relationship, there are few things more intoxicating or more highly anticipated than the first kiss.

And yet, if you've been in a relationship for a long time, maybe you're even married and have kids, somehow kissing can become something you both forget to do.

No matter how long we've been with someone, we continue to need reassurance that we are loved and wanted. And kissing is a small yet magical act that can make people feel closer and happier—it triggers hormones involved in stress relief as well as feelings of bondedness.

So don't forget to give your partner sincere and loving kisses, not just during sex—you can share a tender kiss whenever the opportunity arises for a quiet moment together (consensually, of course!).

FINGERING AND HAND JOBS

Q How can I use my hands to provide pleasure?

Many people's first sexual experiences involve touching each other's genitals with the hand or fingers—fingering, hand jobs, whatever you'd like to call it. Yet, it hardly gets talked about, even in the context of sex education. Manual stimulation is pretty underrated in my opinion—it has the potential to be uniquely pleasurable—because your hands and fingers have the ability to make movements with considerably more precision and range than your genitals!

It's important to make sure your hands are clean and that your nails are short and blunt. Some people even use disposable latex gloves—this is particularly helpful for anal fingering, as even if you're very careful to ensure your hands are clean before you begin, you don't want bacteria from the anus to transfer via your fingers to other parts of the body such as the vagina.

Using lube to moisten your fingers or palm before caressing a vulva, penis, or anus is likely to make things feel much, much more comfortable and fun. In fact, attempting to insert a dry finger inside the vagina or anus can feel very uncomfortable. Lube is your friend.

I love fingering my partner's vagina but I don't think I'm any good at it. How do I do it right? – *Samuel*

Many vulva-owners enjoy the sensation of a finger rubbing the clitoris, as well as the sensation of fingering against the upper wall of the vagina—the wall closest to the belly button—this stimulates the 'G-spot' or clito-urethro-vaginal complex (for more on what exactly the 'G-Spot' is, see page 28). Fingering the vaginal canal can feel especially pleasurable when you're licking or rubbing the external clitoris simultaneously. Start slow and gentle, keeping your movements consistent. Ask your partner to tell you if they'd prefer things faster or more intense!

Do men enjoy hand jobs? I sometimes find it hard to fit a whole penis in my mouth comfortably when giving a blow job. Any tips? Should I use my hands instead? – *Apeksha*

Most penis-owners are well aware that their own hand can be a wonderfully effective pleasure aid—'*apna haath Jagannath*', and all of that. So yup, using your hand to stimulate your partner's penis can certainly provide an exciting and satisfying experience. Using lube makes hand jobs, whether solo or partnered, exceedingly more fun.

Adding your hand to the mix can also make giving a blowjob feel easier and more comfortable, especially if the penis in question is larger than you are able to comfortably accommodate in your mouth. If you combine manual and oral stimulation, you can put a generous amount of lube on your hand and hold and slide your hand along the shaft, while stimulating only the head of the penis with your mouth.

ORAL SEX

Is it weird that I enjoy giving my partner a blowjob? I feel like it's almost taboo to admit as a woman that you like giving blowjobs. – *Sahitya*

How can I become a master of cunnilingus? I like it, but I'm also just a little intimidated. – *Darren*

I find the idea of oral sex so off-putting. I can't bring myself to put a penis in my mouth or lick someone's butthole, and neither can I fathom letting someone lick my vulva or butt. It just all seems rather gross! – *Harpreet*

The mouth and tongue are incredible organs capable of a range of movement and sensation that can be extremely pleasurable indeed. But many of us are also far more squeamish about what we're willing to put in our mouths as compared to what we're willing to touch with our fingers or even our genitals. So while most people seem very curious about oral sex, many are understandably also disgusted by the idea. And perhaps alongside the fact that it can feel amazing, it's in the overcoming of this sense of disgust that lies its appeal.

As Alain De Botton expertly points out in a video titled 'The Philosophy of Oral Sex', which you can watch on *The School of Life* YouTube channel, what makes any erotic act exciting is the fact that these acts could seem disgusting out of context or with a person you don't desire. But in the right context, with someone you adore, that disgust can be replaced by intense arousal and a profound sense of acceptance.

According to Botton, that willingness and enthusiasm from someone you like, to kiss and lick and suck your genitals—to celebrate and shower affection on even the parts of you that you yourself are probably conditioned to be somewhat repulsed or embarrassed by—appeals to our fundamental human need to be wanted and accepted just as we are.

I would agree.

But, as I keep saying, as with any sexual act, oral sex too is not something you should ever feel pressured into giving or receiving. Its whole appeal lies in enthusiastic and mutual consent. If you're not comfortable with oral sex at all, that's fine! As always, don't feel compelled to do anything you don't want to do.

If you are into it, don't hesitate to demonstrate your enthusiasm. It can be so incredibly arousing to witness your partner take pleasure in giving you pleasure!

In case **oral-sex terminology** is confusing to you, here's a quick break down: 'blowjob' is the colloquial term for oral stimulation of the penis. A more formal term for blowjob is 'fellatio'. 'Pussy licking' and 'eating pussy' are colloquialisms for oral stimulation of the vulva, which is an act usually focused on the clitoris. The more formal term for this is 'cunnilingus'.

'Giving head' and 'going down on' someone, are other slang terms for oral sex. 'Annilingus', 'rimming', 'rim job' and 'eating ass' all refer to oral stimulation of the anal region. I think that has us covered on the oral sex vocabulary front. Delicious!

Q How do you have oral sex safely?

Sexually transmitted infections, including human papillomavirus (HPV) and herpes, can be transmitted via oral sex. So if you and your partner haven't been tested for STIs, you should consider using condoms during blowjobs, and dental dams during cunnilingus and anilingus. (For more on how to use protection during oral sex, turn to the section on safer sex on page 124)

Q Is it okay to swallow semen and vaginal fluids?

As we've just covered, if you and your partner haven't been tested for STIs, it's best to use a condom or a dental dam during oral sex, in which case you're not going to need to either spit or swallow any fluids because a condom will collect semen, and a dental dam would prevent vaginal fluids from entering your mouth.

If you've ascertained that STIs are not a concern, and you're simply curious about whether there are any other side effects to ingesting semen or vaginal fluids, then the answer is, nope—semen and vaginal fluids will simply be digested!

Q Is it better to spit or swallow when giving a blowjob?

If you and your partner have been tested, and STIs are not a concern, then it totally depends on how comfortable you feel about spitting and/or swallowing. If, for whatever reason, you're not comfortable with swallowing, or even spitting for that matter, just say so. Your partner can ejaculate elsewhere or into a tissue.

If you are both comfortable with oral sex and swallowing, then that's something you can both enjoy as part of the experience. If you prefer to spit it out, spit it out. It's up to you to decide what your preferences are.

It's common courtesy to inform your partner before you ejaculate when receiving a blowjob so they can decide how they'd like to go about it.

Q Should I worry about how I taste and smell down there?

This is perhaps one of the most common questions around oral sex that I get asked, especially by women.

At the risk of making a generalization, I think people with vulvas worry too much about this, and people with penises sometimes don't worry enough.

Before any sexual activity, it's great to have a shower. Wash your vulva (external genitals only, not inside the vaginal canal), wash your penis, wash your balls, wash your pubes, your butt, your underarms. Who doesn't love a nice shower! Enjoy the process. Showering before getting naked, if you can, is a nice thing to do—whatever your gender. Showering together can be fun too!

Basically, as long as you generally maintain your personal hygiene, there's no need to worry about what you taste and smell like. Your genitals are not going to taste or smell like strawberries or roses and it's absurd to expect them to.

Even right after a shower, the genitals may have a bit of their own unique scent and taste. It's not a 'bad' smell or taste; it just is what it is. *A huge part of being able to enjoy sexual intimacy is getting over one's squeamishness around the body in its natural state.*

Q Do I have to wax or shave my pubic hair if I want to receive oral sex?

It's worth remembering that oral sex has been around far longer than the trend of pubic hair waxing.

Porn has certainly impacted how we think bodies ought to look like during sex—and that's perhaps partly why more and more people seem to experience this pressure to get rid of their pubes.

But, as I've covered earlier in the section on the body, pubes exist for a reason: they protect against friction and infection. There are no health benefits to waxing or shaving them off. It's simply an aesthetic choice and depends entirely on your own preference.

Q How do I initiate oral sex?

If you'd like to initiate oral sex, it's usually a good idea to offer it first. In sex, as in life, reciprocity is usually much appreciated. But don't assume; *ask*. Ask your partner for their consent, even to give them oral. Ask if they'd be interested in giving you oral.

Resorting to non-verbal moves to ask for oral sex, particularly in a first-time hook-up or with someone you don't already have exceptional communication and very clearly understood boundaries with, is a terrible idea.

In fact, let's talk about the problematic '**blowjob head push**'. This is particularly common in heterosexual encounters, where the man tries to initiate oral sex by pushing down the woman's head mid-make out, sort of physically directing her head to his crotch instead of respectfully and clearly communicating his desire verbally first.

Unless you know your partner very well and they have explicitly indicated they like having their head pushed, *do not* just push down someone's head when you want a blowjob. Because this registers as a demand for oral sex, not an ask. It becomes much harder to willingly give consent because, instead of initiating a verbal discussion of consent, you are literally pushing them, and in order to decline, the person not only has to say no, they also have to literally resist your pressure.

Even if the person was quite excited about giving oral sex, when you do this, it is likely to be a major buzzkill. At best, the person doing the head pushing seems entitled and creepy; at worst, it can feel like something rather close to sexual assault.

Oral sex can be a lot of fun, but only when it's done willingly. So *talk about it*. And make your partner's sense of safety and pleasure as much of a priority as your own. Seek each other's consent. And honour each other's boundaries. If someone says 'no' to something, respect that too. *Respectful, clear communication is key.*

Q How do I get good at oral sex?

I do believe that, ultimately, the best way to figure out how to make your partner feel good is to ask them what feels good. Being able to communicate honestly and actively with your partner about sex is arguably the most effective thing you can do to become a better lover.

It can also be a huge turn-on to see your partner enjoying themselves with you, whether giving or receiving oral; so when you're enjoying yourself, don't hesitate to let your enjoyment be known!

And remember that you can also use your hands along with your mouth.

While a lot of people want to know 'how to give good oral sex', especially for vulva-owners, getting more comfortable *receiving* oral sex is also something worth thinking about.

For example, for many vulva-owners, receiving oral sex comes with thoughts like *'Gosh, I hope they're okay down there'*, *'I hope it's not too smelly or gross'*, or *'Am I taking too long?'* which can really get in the way of enjoying the experience.

Whether giving or receiving, try to be present in the moment, communicate with your partner about what feels good, and really enjoy every sensation.

And I know I keep saying this, but the key to a pleasurable sexual experience is consent. And consent is an ongoing process. Check in with your partner not just before the act, but throughout the act.

As I mentioned, even something as seemingly small as putting your hands on their head while they're at it is something you should ask about first.

HOW TO LICK A PUSSY

While you can kiss any part of the vulva if that's what you and your partner like, most people are likely to prefer that you focus your energies on the clitoris. You can gently part the labia or vaginal lips using your hands, or ask your partner to do that, so you have easier access to the clitoris.

Different people may enjoy different intensities of stimulation, so it's a good idea to start as gently as if you were licking honey off a flower petal, and you can work your way up to something like the enthusiasm of a puppy licking an ice-cream cone.

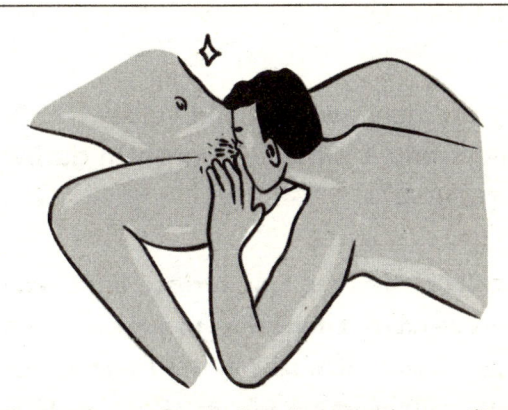

As with any form of oral sex, with cunnilingus too, you can use your lips, tongue, mouth; you can lick, kiss, suck, flick and tickle—but you might want to pick your technique and stick with it for a bit before doing something different instead of switching things up in very rapid succession. *For many people, a single movement repeated consistently is more effective than a jumble of different types of moves.*

Since clitorises and penises are actually very similar to each other, here's a question for penis-owners: doesn't that description of how to lick a clitoris sound like it would work great for a blowjob too?

These are just some ideas to get you started. Ultimately, only you and your partner know exactly how each of you likes things. So the best and most important tip of all is: *communicate*!

P.S. Take your time. There's nothing quite like a lover who is generous with time spent on oral, and eager to incorporate feedback. It just hits different when someone seems to genuinely love doing it.

VAGINAL SEX

Q Why do many women and vulva-owners find it difficult to orgasm during intercourse?

I orgasm really easily when I masturbate, but intercourse gets me there so rarely. I don't want to make my boyfriend feel inadequate, so I often fake it. But I wish I could tell him it's not really working for me so we could switch things up and ensure I have more fun. Any tips for how to have an orgasm during penetrative sex, for people with vulvas? – *Dimple*

Why do women fake orgasm? I'm pretty sure my girlfriend is faking it when we have sex, and I appreciate that this is probably because she doesn't want to hurt my feelings, but I genuinely want to learn how to give her pleasure so she doesn't have to pretend. What can I do to make sex actually enjoyable for her? – *Saptak*

I touched upon this in the section on clitoral anatomy (see page 26), but in case you need a recap: for many people with vulvas, penetration is not the most reliable route to orgasm. Some amount of external clitoral stimulation is also required.

But sex continues to be defined—particularly in heterosexual relationships—as penis-in-vagina penetration.

The necessary sequence tends to be: erection, penetration, ejaculation—sex revolves around the penis and ends when he comes. Clitoral stimulation is too often relegated to the realm of the optional—it's considered 'foreplay'—instead of a vital sex act in and of itself.

A lot of men mistakenly seem to think that sex is about jackhammering a penis as fast as possible into a vagina. But sex is so much more than that, and going straight from taking your clothes off to jackhammering is almost never a good idea. It can even be really uncomfortable or painful. It usually takes a little time for our bodies to feel sufficiently relaxed and aroused.

Unfortunately, too often for straight women, sex can just sort of feel like you're serving as a vessel into which the man is masturbating—it's no fun having sex with someone who doesn't know or care about your pleasure and is in a hurry to satisfy himself and get it over with.

And so, for many women, faking it often simply seems like the least awkward way to end sex when it's clear that orgasms (for them) are not on the menu. I myself have faked orgasms because I didn't want to hurt a partner's feelings, I didn't want to seem like I was sexually inept, or because it seemed like the easiest, quickest and safest way to end the sex. It's no fun to think about that, but there it is.

If we understand that sex can be so much more than just penetration, as well as acknowledge how central to the pleasure of vulva-owners the clitoris can be; if we give equal priority to the pleasure of people of all genders, and become more comfortable giving and receiving feedback in bed; if we stop attaching our egos to how well we think we are able to individually 'perform' sexually and, instead, see sex as a shared experience and an opportunity to learn about each other's pleasure; if we can get better at making each other feel comfortable and safe expressing ourselves in bed, not only when we enjoy something but even when something isn't working for us, we're all likely to have far more mutually joyful experiences.

Sex can be a lot of fun! But there's more to sex than just thrusting as fast and hard as possible. Slow down, explore, savour, play, be present, take your time!

Remember: Most vulva owners don't orgasm from penetration alone. Clitoral stimulation is also required!

External clitoral stimulation alone can result in orgasm for many vulva-owners; clitoral + vaginal stimulation together can feel amazing for many vulva-owners, but penetration alone does not result in orgasm for the majority of people with vulvas.

(Of course, everyone's pleasure has unique specificities, and some people with vulvas may indeed enjoy how penetration feels on its own—but these are some general overarching insights that are worth keeping in mind.)

Once you grasp this, it's actually pretty easy to navigate pleasure for vulvas—clitoral stimulation or a combination of clitoral and vaginal stimulation can be achieved using hands, mouth, toys or a combination thereof and, in fact, it can even be achieved during vaginal intercourse.

Positions to Try

If you'd like to explore how penis-in-vagina sex can become more pleasurable for both partners, here are some positions that enable adequate friction on the external clitoris alongside penetration.

The **'woman on top' or 'cowgirl'** position is often a favourite to maximize pleasure during vaginal intercourse because it allows the person with the vulva to have more control over the movements, making it easier for them to ensure that their external clitoris is also getting some stimulation—typically against the partner's pubic mound or lower abdomen.

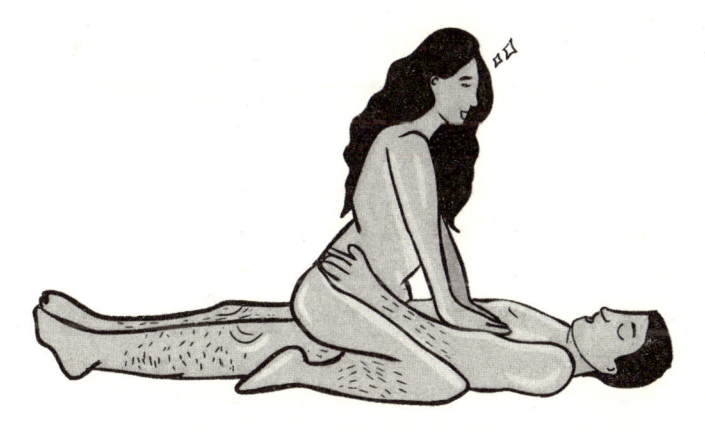

Another position that lends itself to simultaneous clitoral and vaginal stimulation is the **Coital Alignment Technique** or

CAT. It's a variation on the standard 'missionary' sex position, tweaked to ensure that the clitoris is no longer ignored.

Instead of the typical in-and-out thrusting motion, penetration can take the form of a deeper rocking/grinding/rubbing motion—a rocking up and down instead of a thrusting in and out—with both partners pressing up against each other. This often allows for adequate, sustained clitoral stimulation alongside penetration.

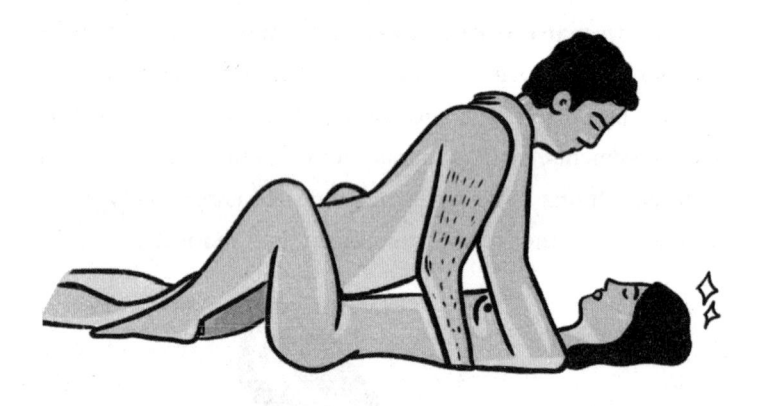

Basically, if partners can place themselves in such a way so as to try to ensure that the vulva-owner's clitoris can rub against the partner's body during penetration, it's more likely to be a satisfying experience for both people instead of for just the penis-owner.

Using lube on the clitoris and on the section of the partner's lower belly or pelvic region against which it is rubbing ensures greater comfort and pleasure.

While often suggested in the context of heterosexual penis-in-vagina sex, in fact these positions can also be explored by partners who both have vulvas, with either partner using a **strap-on dildo** (see page 217).

Q What is squirting?

Sometimes when the sex is really great, and often when I'm masturbating with my toys, if I get that perfect combination of clitoral and vaginal stimulation together, I think I squirt—it's almost as if I need to pee but can't quite control myself—but it also feels different from peeing because it's really pleasurable—almost like I can't contain my pleasure and I'm ejaculating! Is this normal? – *Leanne*

Squirting is the involuntary expulsion of liquid from the urethra by people with vulvas during sexual activity. The liquid may contain traces of urine as well as a thicker liquid called female ejaculate, produced by the Skene's glands (also called the female prostate) which are a pair of little glands located on each side of the urethral opening.

While some people experience squirting during sex or masturbation, it's worth knowing that in porn, squirting is often artificially created.

If you squirt, cool! Feel free to uninhibitedly enjoy this aspect of your body and pleasure. If you've never squirted, though, that's fine too! Neither is it something to worry about if it happens, nor is it something to feel pressured to try to do.

> ### WHAT TO FOLLOW
>
> If you're interested in learning more about how people with vulvas experience orgasm, I highly recommend subscribing to **omgyes.com**. It is a fantastic in-depth study that explores how hundreds of vulva-owners navigate and experience pleasure. It has incredible video demonstrations and interviews with real people of diverse ethnicities and age groups, as well as interactive exercises that allow you to explore and practice a variety of techniques using the touch screen of your smartphone or tablet. It is *truly* remarkable.

Q How can I last longer in bed?

When it comes to the concerns of people with penises on the other hand, what I get asked most with regard to intercourse is, 'How can I last longer?'

I'm not a fan of climax delay condoms and sprays as they typically contain ingredients that work by numbing the skin, and can therefore limit sensation for both partners. There are also all kinds of tablets and pills out there promising 'virility', 'vigour', and 'stamina', but too often, their efficacy is dubious, and I wouldn't recommend taking any medication without consulting a doctor.

But here's a technique that requires no medication, is free, and can be a lot of fun: Edging! It's also sometimes called the 'start-stop' technique.

Q What is edging?

Edging is the sexual practice of delaying your orgasm so you can prolong the time until climax. While it can be practised by anyone of any gender, it is often suggested as a technique for people with penises to 'last longer', as premature ejaculation tends to be a common concern among penis-owners. (For more on premature ejaculation, see page 92)

By pausing or switching things up when you feel yourself approaching orgasm, and repeating this a few times, you can keep enjoying solo or partnered sexual activity for a longer duration before ultimately climaxing.

ANAL SEX

The idea of anal play excites me but I literally don't know anything about it. Like where do I start, how does it work? What do I need to know? What if there's poop? – *Josey*

Many people feel squeamish at the mention of anal sex—butt, butt, butt, of course, many of us are also very titillated by the prospect.

The Importance of Condoms and Lube

Whatever your gender or sexual orientation, it's important to note that *the anus is not self-lubricating*. So before you begin exploring the region, whether solo or with a partner, you're going to need lube. Lots of it.

While you can't get pregnant from anal play, you can contract sexually transmitted infections—both from genital and oral contact with the anus—so condoms and dental dams are your friends. *Anal sex without condoms and condom-compatible lube is not a good idea.*

Q Will there be poop?

Many people are worried about the possibility of encountering poop when exploring the anal region, but it's not like poop is just hanging out there all the time. If you've already pooped that day and you also washed your butt again before sex, things can be pretty fresh and clean, and mess-free.

Still, encountering poop remains a risk you take when you embark on this journey, so it's a possibility you've just got to wrap your head around if you'd like to explore butt stuff. If it does happen, what can you do? Go wash it off.

Anal Fingering

Adding some anal play to your masturbation routine—just by using your own finger (and some lube)—is a simple way to begin your anal explorations because that way you're in control and you can figure out what feels good and what doesn't.

If you'd like to attempt anal play with a partner, as with any sex act, consent and communication are absolutely vital. Talk about it first.

Whether with a partner or solo, and no matter your gender, *it's best to begin exploring anal play after you're already feeling very relaxed and aroused.*

Rimming

The technical term for oral–anal stimulation is **annilingus**, and the slang term for it is **rimming** or if you'd like to get straight to the point, 'eating ass'.

Licking the skin between the genitals and the anus (that stretch is called the **perineum**), and then moving to licking the external area around the anus, can be an especially intimate and exciting way to explore the region.

Using your hands to gently part your lover's butt cheeks makes rimming much easier to execute.

For many people—for reasons similar to the ones Alain De Botton listed on the appeal of oral sex—rimming can be an especially erotically charged and pleasurable experience because of the profound sense of acceptance that being willing to perform the act on one another would seem to suggest. However, it's best to use a **dental dam** for safer annilingus (see page 124).

Anal fingering and rimming are a gentle way to ease into anal play—and for many, this is the extent of anal play that they wish to incorporate into their sexual life, whether solo or partnered.

It's really up to you or you and your partner to decide what you are comfortable with and there's obviously no pressure to do anything you don't want to.

Anal Sex

You might not manage to have full-blown penetrative anal sex the very first time you try anal play with a partner. It often takes some preparation, and it isn't meant to be painful. So take your time to ease into it, and be sure to use condoms and LOTS of lube. You need to be careful in order to avoid injury.

Before you get to attempting anal penetration with a penis or dildo, it can help to first get totally comfortable stimulating the area with a **butt plug** (see page 218). You can even get sets of butt plugs that are in a gradation of sizes so that you can gradually work your way from the smallest one to slightly bigger ones as you get more comfortable.

If you're ever switching between anal and vaginal stimulation, change your condom and wash your hands. You don't want bacteria from the anus entering the vagina as it can cause vaginal infections.

Another thing to note: Butt plugs and prostate massagers have flared bases for a reason. You never want to use any toy or object without a flared base or handle inside the anus because it could be sucked in too far and then difficult to remove. Unlike the vagina, where you can go no further than the cervix, the anus has no barrier preventing an object from going inside the body—so only use toys that are specifically designed for anal play.

Is anal sex more pleasurable for men than for women?
– Raj

Anal sex can be pleasurable for people of all genders, but it can be especially enjoyable for people with **prostates** (usually people with penises have prostates). Many cishet men are unaware that they have this erogenous zone (see page 97), and often their internalized homophobia prevents them from exploring it.

That said, some people like anal sex and some people don't, and that's fine. Whatever your gender and sexual orientation, you get to determine your own personal sexual preferences and boundaries.

I'm a straight man, but I'm turned on by the idea of receiving anal stimulation. Is that normal or is something wrong with me? *– Ritwik*

A lot of straight men seem excited at the prospect of providing anal penetration to a woman, yet they have this homophobic idea that being open to receiving any sort of anal play would make them 'gay', and that being gay is 'not normal'. Firstly, there should be no place for homophobia in our lives. Secondly, anal play is not solely or inherently gay. It doesn't matter what your sexual orientation is—there are straight people who enjoy anal play and there are gay people who don't. Fantasizing about or participating in anal play is not something that is necessarily determined by or determining of your gender, sexuality or sexual orientation. Your body and your pleasure are yours to explore and enjoy however you choose solo, and with the consent of your partner during partnered sexual experiences.

Pegging

Pegging usually refers to a woman wearing a strap-on dildo to stimulate the anus of a male partner. It's a sex act that subverts traditional power dynamics and challenges the widely held heteronormative notion that a man is the *penetrator* and a woman, *penetrated.*

However, pegging can also more generally be used to describe anal penetration with a strap-on dildo by participants of any gender identity and sexual orientation.

If my DMs are anything to go by, given the newfound prominence of the term in internet culture and porn, more people seem curious about pegging than ever before. However, it seems that for many, the curiosity is laced with shame and disgust. As we've already touched upon—for many people, and especially for cishet men, anal play remains a major taboo, largely because of society's overarching homophobia and misogyny. It's worth thinking about why we feel the way we do about certain sexual acts versus others, and begin to unpack any unexamined prejudices.

Consent and communication are essential in exploring whether pegging might be something you and your partner want to try. You're also definitely going to need lube. And a strap-on dildo.

AROUSAL

Q What's the most powerful sexual organ?

This may come as a surprise, but it isn't the penis. It isn't even the clitoris or anus. It's the brain! Sex is not a mindless activity—far from it. The brain orchestrates the sexual response cycle and facilitates everything from desire to arousal to orgasm.

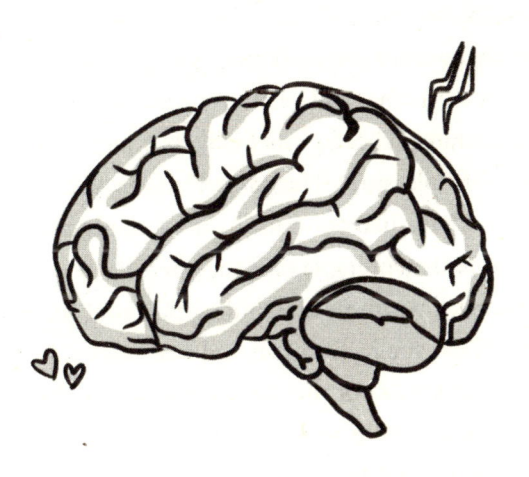

So if you're wondering how to have better sex—you might want to think about what's going on between your ears rather than just what's going on in your pants. The mind matters just as much as the body, if not more.

A lot of the time, advice for better sex is oriented around the physical or mechanical stuff only—try this or that position; use this or that sex technique or pleasure product, etc. But, in fact, some of the most effective things you can do for better sex have to do with the mental and emotional realm rather than just the physical. Being present and focused, feeling relaxed, feeling uninhibited and enthusiastic, experiencing heightened empathy, being open to expressing vulnerability and connection, communicating and listening, flirting, banter—all of this can really elevate your sexual experiences.

It's kind of sad that we've come to associate the mental and emotional aspects of intimacy with a sense of burdensome commitment or obligation. So often, with casual sex, it's like let's just pretend we have nothing going on in our heads or hearts, fuck each other and get it over with. But even in a casual sexual encounter, 'clicking' mentally, not just physically, can really amplify pleasure! That doesn't mean you have to get married and have babies—but it can certainly mean a more pleasurable and memorable time together!

It's also well worth understanding that your mental health can impact how you feel sexually and vice versa.

Your brain sends out the signals that radiate through your central nervous system to trigger symptoms of sexual arousal in your genitals, and the pleasure that you experience during a positive sexual experience, is manifest in the release of neurochemicals in the brain.

Common mental health issues like depression and anxiety, as well as the medications used to treat these, tend to impact those same neurochemicals. How you are feeling mentally, and how you are feeling sexually, are likely to have a powerful and intimate correlation.

Just as pleasurable sexual experiences, whether solo or partnered, can have many mental health benefits, sexual trauma can adversely impact your mental health.

Similarly, if you're in a great space mentally, it's likely to have a positive impact on your relationship with your sexuality, while struggles with your mental health can sometimes adversely impact your sexual life.

> **Q** Why do we sometimes get an erection/experience wetness even when we are not aroused, while at other times struggle to get an erection/experience wetness even in a sexual situation?

A rather inconvenient truth about our bodies (true for penis-owners and vulva-owners alike) is that it is possible to sometimes have an erection/experience wetness even when you're not actually turned on. And it's also possible to feel aroused yet not get an erection/experience wetness. A seeming mismatch between your mental experience of arousal and the expected genital response is a phenomenon called '**arousal non-concordance**', most famously described in Emily Nagoski's masterful book *Come As You Are* (which you absolutely must read). Arousal non-concordance is extremely common.

It's also worth noting that while we're told that 'penises get hard' and 'vaginas get wet' when aroused, clits can have erections too, and penises can get wet too! Just as the penis can become engorged with blood when aroused to form an erection, even the clitoris can become engorged with blood when aroused. And just as the vagina can produce lubrication or wetness, the penis can release precum—that's the penis's way of getting wet!

So, both wetness and hardness can occur during arousal for both penis- and vulva-owners. However, that doesn't mean that these bodily functions always indicate arousal, or that their absence necessarily indicates the absence of arousal.

Arousal non-concordance is so common, in fact, that we're all likely to experience it on occasion, and it's generally nothing to worry about, even though to many it can seem rather confusing, and often leaves one feeling embarrassed. It's just the body being the body, doing its own thing in its intriguing, wonderful and sometimes seemingly eccentric way.

It's also why it's so *very* important to actually talk about how you're feeling with your partner, rather than assume consent or assume that they're not attracted to you simply based on how their bodies seem to be responding.

Moaning

As a woman, do I have to moan during sex? I worry my partner will think I'm boring or that I'm not enjoying myself if I don't make some sounds during sex. – *Manasvi*

Is it okay for men to moan during sex? I tend to moan when I'm about to cum but my girlfriend always looks at me weird if I moan loudly, so I stop myself. – *Bijoy*

Sometimes I moan just to get the sex done with—I think it turns my partner on to hear me moan, he's more likely to come quickly and it's just an easy way to move things along without hurting his feelings so I can be done too when I'm not really feeling like I'm going to orgasm any time soon. But then other times when I'm really horny and really enjoying the sex, I feel that moaning actually helps me get more into it too—like I might start off by sort of performing the moans but the sound of my own moaning and the heavy breathing really gets me more aroused! So is performative moaning good or bad? Help me figure this out! – *Mariana*

The younger me thought that I *had to* moan in bed, even if the sex didn't actually feel that great, because if porn is anything to go by, it seemed like moaning is something women who are 'good in bed' always do during sex. Many women feel this sort of gendered expectation to moan during sex—whether or not they are actually enjoying themselves.

I realize now that most porn is a performance, skewed to cater to the male gaze, and most of those moans are just actors doing their job. I'm also now much less interested in feigning pleasure because I've learnt that communicating with my partner and telling them what I actually like is much more likely to result in more pleasurable sex for me. While if I moan when a partner does something I'm not actually enjoying, not only do I have to pretend to enjoy it this once, they're likely to do the same thing again and again—after all, by moaning, I've made them think I enjoy it!

From faking orgasms to moaning and making facial expressions in the ways that we assume we 'ought to', based on porn, to feigning comfort in uncomfortable positions because we want to please our partner or seem 'good in bed' to them, performative sex is something that people of any gender may find themselves doing.

But for women it tends to be a majority experience, thanks to the combination of mainstream porn being the major visual reference point for sex with its overemphasis on men's pleasure, the socialization and depiction of women in society as somehow responsible for keeping their partners/husbands happy no matter whether they are happy themselves, and a lack of access to accurate information about how our bodies work in relation to pleasure. Too often we moan only because we think we have to, or because it helps get unsatisfying sex over with.

But no one 'has to' moan during sex. If you're doing it only because you think you have to, and it's not something you enjoy, know that it's absolutely okay to stop doing it.

If you're moaning to get unsatisfying sex over with, why not take the time to understand your pleasure and communicate what you enjoy with your partner so that the sex can become more genuinely satisfying for you as well?

Ironically, while many women seem to feel a pressure to moan during sex, some men seem to feel like they have to stop themselves from moaning with pleasure because it's 'not manly'. That's the problem with rigidly binary gender stereotypes—they constantly get in the way of all of us being able to actually be ourselves.

For people of all genders, feelings of pleasure can indeed elicit moans. Many people are also excited by the very act and sound of moaning, be it their own, or their partner's moans. If you're moaning because you're aroused, or because it arouses you to moan, or because it excites you to excite your partner, then no matter your gender, by all means, moan away!

On the other hand, some people feel more comfortable being quiet during sex, or don't really feel the need to moan. Again—totally fine, no matter your gender.

There's no pressure to moan if you don't want to, and there's no shame in moaning if you do. You get to decide what floats your boat!

Dirty Talk

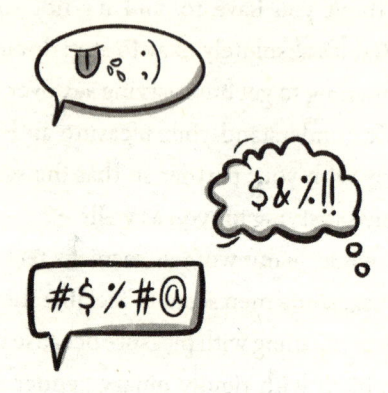

Is it weird that I like saying really explicit things sometimes in bed? I like telling my boyfriend stuff like 'I want to be your dirty little slut' or 'I want to put your rock-hard dick inside my soft, wet pussy' when we're having really passionate sex. He dare not call me any degrading names, that's personally a boundary for me—but when I'm extremely turned on, I like saying this stuff about myself, and I like it when we talk about sex in a really explicit way too. Funny thing is, I am such a prude about talking about sex otherwise. But when I'm super super aroused, I feel like talking dirty really takes things to another level of pleasure. Am I weird for liking this? I mean, people say men like dirty talk, but is it weird that I'm a woman and I like it? – *Shivi*

In the right circumstances—with a partner with whom consent and mutual respect are already well-established—dirty talk can be incredibly arousing for many people, of all genders.

After all, arousal starts in the brain—and erotic communication can enhance sexual arousal and pleasure for many.

Some people may enjoy dirty talk because it's an expression of uninhibitedness—being able to say things to each other that you wouldn't be able to say out loud anywhere else can be very titillating.

It may also feel like a marker of how close and vulnerable and unjudging you're able to be with each other: that you can trust each other enough to explore your 'wilder', 'freakier' sides together can feel thrilling!

Dirty talk may also allow for partners to verbally articulate fantasies they may not have the ability or intention to act on—simply talking about them can be hot in itself—intensifying arousal and pleasure during sex.

Some may find that dirty talk helps them get out of their own head and feel more 'in the moment'. For others, dirty talk may feel enjoyably over-the-top and humorous—it may provide a moment of lightness and laughter.

But, of course, all of that said, some people may not like dirty talk at all. Some may find it insulting or uncomfortable or overwhelming to participate in—and that's totally okay too.

Everyone's sexual preferences and boundaries are different, which is why it's so important to communicate about whether or not each of you is into it or would be open to exploring something, before trying it out during sex.

So if you're curious to try dirty talk with your partner in bed, be sure to discuss it beforehand. As I keep saying, consent and communication are fundamental prerequisites for pleasure.

LUBE

What is lube exactly? There seem to be quite a few types—how do I know which one I should use? – *Hitesh*

Is it really safe to put lube inside the vagina? What about using coconut oil or body lotion as lube—is that okay? – *Sharda*

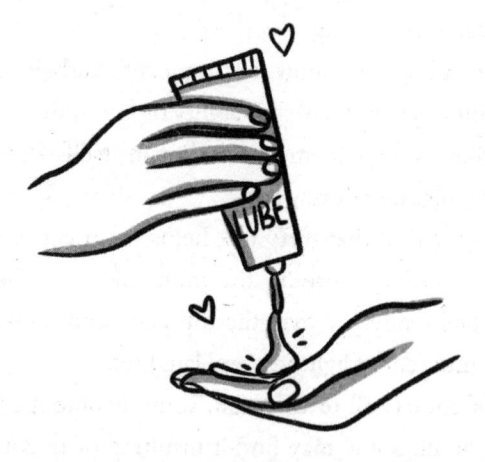

I've mentioned lube quite a few times in this book, and I really do think of it as one of the unsung heroes of better sex for everyone. I only started using lube in my late twenties, but I wish I'd discovered it sooner. It's hard to imagine sex or masturbation without it now. It can make everything so much more comfortable and fun!

A 'lube' (short for lubricant) is a substance that reduces friction and makes things move more smoothly.

You've likely seen huge billboards at petrol pumps advertising lube for car and bike engines—if only sexual lube were as widely available! While, of course, they have totally different ingredients and cannot be used interchangeably (you never want to put engine oil on your genitals, obvs!), the principle is the same. Just as car and bike lubes are designed to make vehicles work with less friction and wear and tear, a sexual lubricant (available at pharmacies and online) allows for things to be much more slippery-slidey, wet, smooth and pain-free in bed.

Pain during sex is often the result of excessive friction and insufficient lubrication—and here's where lube can really help. But even in general, lube just tends to elevate the pleasure and make sex more fun. And, as I said a little while ago, it can make masturbation feel even better too.

Many people think lube is only for vaginal dryness. And while it can certainly help with that, lube can be used on many other parts of the body to great effect too!

You can lube up a finger before touching a vagina or anus; you can lube up your hand before rubbing a penis; you can put lube on your clitoris and on your partner's lower belly during intercourse to ensure movements feel smoother if you like rubbing and grinding your pelvic region against their body to achieve simultaneous clitoral stimulation alongside penetration.

Most of us already do this stuff using saliva—so even if we haven't thought about it, in fact, most of us already recognize the need for additional slipperiness. Lube does a way better job than saliva, and it's also safer! Some STIs, including herpes and HPV, can be transmitted to the genitals via saliva. You can also get a vaginal infection because the bacteria and enzymes in saliva can sometimes disrupt the vaginal ecosystem. Also, saliva isn't as effective as lube because it isn't as slippery, and it dries faster.

You can put lube on your toys; on your genitals or any other body part, or on your condom; on the rim of a menstrual cup for easier insertion—there are many great ways to use lube.

Q Which lube should you use?

There are three main types of personal lubricants available: water-based, oil-based, and silicone-based.

A **water-based sexual lube** is a good place to start if you've never used lube before and you're wondering which one to buy. Some lubes have a thinner, more liquidy consistency, while others have a thicker, more gel-like consistency—you could try a few different ones to figure out which you like best. Water-based lube is generally the most easily available type of lube at pharmacies. It's compatible with all types of condoms and sex toys, it's easy to wash off, and it won't stain your sheets.

Oil-based and silicone-based sexual lubes dry less quickly than water-based ones, and therefore require less reapplication—so many people like these as well. They tend to have a slicker texture than water-based lubes.

Silicone-based lubes, in particular, feel quite unique because, unlike water or oil, silicone does not get absorbed by the skin. A good silicone lube can have a very pleasant, silky feel. It's particularly great for anal play as silicone lube is extremely slippery and doesn't dry out—and the anus produces no lubrication of its own, so this is very helpful! It's also great for sex in the shower or bathtub—it stays put even when exposed to water.

Silicone-based lubes are compatible with condoms—in fact, most condoms come pre-lubricated with a silicone-based lube. However, *silicone-based lube is generally not recommended with silicone sex toys*, as the silicones can bond together and transfer between products—basically, over time, this can sometimes cause the silicone material of the toy to break down.

Oil-based lubes feel, well, oily. Which can be really nice too—there's a delicious warmth to oil, and it's especially suitable if you also like giving each other body massages during sex. Pure coconut oil is an excellent lube—however, it's important to make sure that it really is *pure* coconut oil. Many of the hair oil brands that sell 'coconut oil' have other ingredients in there too, that are not intended for internal use. Use pure coconut oil or a coconut oil-based sexual lube rather than coconut oil-based skincare or haircare products.

However, bear in mind that *oil-based lubes can cause condoms to tear*, as oil can cause latex to break down. So remember never to use an oil-based lube with condoms. It's great for masturbation, and for partnered sex where you've both established that neither STIs nor accidental pregnancy is a concern, and therefore there is no longer a need to use condoms.

If you've never used lube before, a water-based lube is a good place to begin your explorations. If you discover that you do enjoy using lube though (and chances are, you will—it's awesome!), it's worth trying out all three types, as each type offers its own unique possibilities for pleasure!

Most general body lotions, cold creams, balms and moisturizers are intended only for external use on the skin and typically have ingredients that aren't safe for internal use. Please don't use these on your genitals—they will most likely cause discomfort. Use a good sexual lube!

SEX TOYS

Q What are sex toys?

Sex toys are products that have been created specifically to provide sexual pleasure! From simple, non-motorized objects, to ones that integrate highly sophisticated technology and design, there are all sorts of sex toys out there for different body parts and different types of stimulation. The universe of sex toys sure is an exciting one!

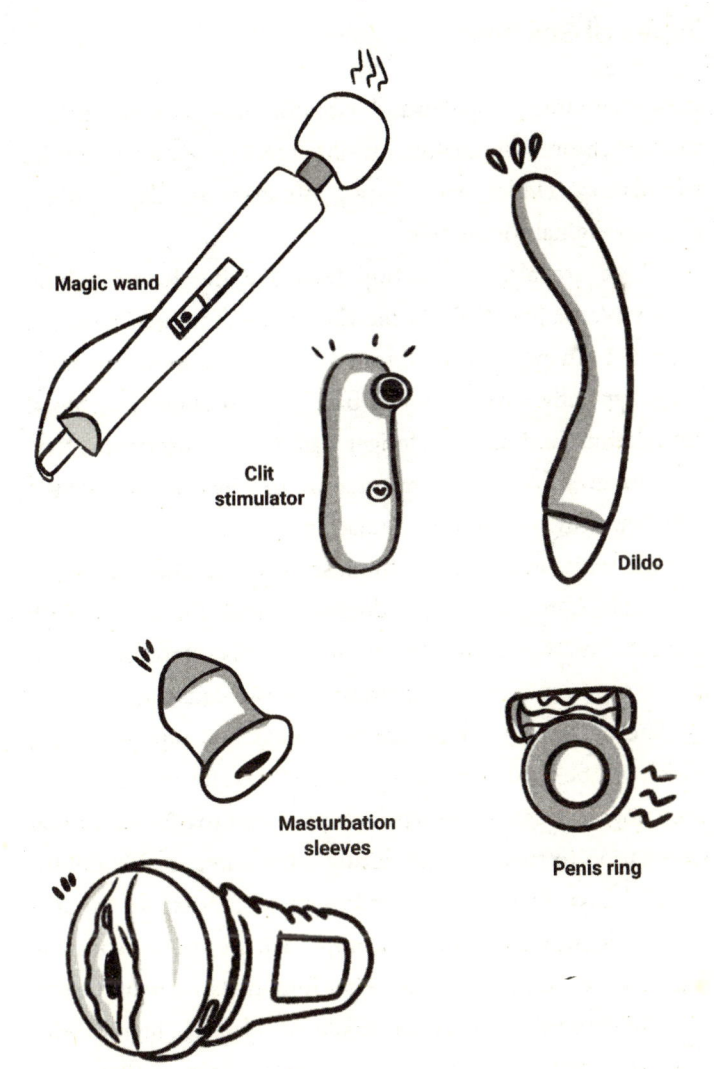

Pleasure

Magic wand

Clit stimulator

Dildo

Masturbation sleeves

Penis ring

Types of Sex Toys

Bullet vibrators, magic-wand vibrators and clitoral suction toys or clitoral stimulators are intended for external clitoral stimulation. Dildos and G-spot vibrators are designed for internal vaginal stimulation.

There are also dual-action toys like the iconic 'rabbit' style vibrator that *Sex and the City* made famous. These can provide both external and internal stimulation simultaneously. They typically have a shorter part that provides the clitoral stimulation, and another longer part that is insertable. New variants even have a clitoral suction arm instead of the little vibrating arm, for clitoral stimulation.

And while many people think sex toys are only for people with vulvas, there are also dozens of toys for people with penises—masturbation sleeves of all kinds—motorized and non-motorized, as well as an array of prostate massagers.

Then there are things like butt plugs and nipple clamps, which can be used by anyone, as well as toys for couples—like cock rings that can be worn by a penis-owner to provide clitoral stimulation to their partner during intercourse; or Bluetooth-enabled toys that allow for partners to participate in each other's pleasure using a mobile app—which can be especially fun for virtual intimacy if you're in a long-distance relationship.

While most sex toys are made of silicone, high-quality glass and steel toys are also a whole universe of their own worth exploring because they can last forever, are very easy to keep clean and also allow for interesting new sensations like temperature play. You can easily warm or cool glass or steel toys by washing them in warm or cold water first. (Btw, in case glass sounds scary, it's good to know that glass toys are made of a special toughened glass that is extremely hard to break and is non-porous.)

How to Choose a Sex Toy

As a 'first' toy, a basic vibrating massager is usually a great bet if you have a vulva—vibrations provide extremely pleasurable clitoral stimulation, and if it has a powerful motor, you don't even have to take your clothes off!

Many people with penises start off with a simple masturbation sleeve as their first toy—they are fun and easy to use—all you need is some lube!

Both these types of toys are also typically affordable and non-intimidating, yet they're highly effective.

That said, do your own research based on your own preferences. Read reviews about the toys that sound exciting to you. If something else sounds like it's more likely to work well for you, go for it! And you can get yourself a whole bunch of different toys over time—many people enjoy using different ones for different types of stimulation. It can be a real *pleasure* to slowly build your own little collection!

Make sure whatever you get yourself is made of a body-safe material, especially if it's an insertable toy—medical grade silicone is much better than most plastics, for example, as it is non-porous and therefore more hygienic.

As I mentioned, it's definitely a good idea to also get yourself lube, as most toys feel much more comfortable and fun when you apply lube when using them.

Keeping your toys clean is important. So choose toys that are waterproof, so you can easily wash them *before* and *after* use. Bonus—you can use them in the shower!

Rechargeable toys tend to be more convenient than battery-operated ones that require you to keep buying and replacing batteries—and they are often of higher quality.

Feel free to use toys together—each toy doesn't have to just be used on its own! You could have a clitoral vibrator and a beautiful glass or steel dildo, for example—they can make a fantastic combination!

If you're sharing toys with multiple partners—make sure to be extra proactive about thoroughly washing your toys before and after use and be sure to use condoms on insertable toys—safety first!

I recently got myself a vibrator, and my partner seems very threatened by it. Can you use sex toys even with your partner, or are they only for masturbation? – *Gayatri*

Sex toys can be wonderful tools, not only for solo pleasure—they can also greatly enhance the experience of partnered sex. They can function as a collaborator rather than some sort of competition to either of you.

A lot of straight men seem to view their partner using their vibrator as some sort of threat—but in fact, vibrators can actually ease a lot of the pressure around 'performance' that men often feel.

Vibrators are uniquely effective at providing clitoral stimulation in particular. They're able to provide a speed and consistency that is hard for a human being to replicate, but that is uniquely effective at delivering orgasms. I think of it this way—there is a technology that exists that stands to make sex more pleasurable—why not embrace it!

Just as an accountant isn't threatened by a calculator but rather uses one to work more efficiently, so, also, sex toys can be terrific pleasure aides without detracting from a partnered experience. I'm a big fan of adding toys to the mix in bed!

What is a strap-on used for? – *Anand*

A strap-on is a sex toy that comprises a harness and a dildo so you can strap it on—hence the name. Strap-ons are perhaps most commonly used when two people with vaginas want to have penetrative sex, such as in a lesbian relationship, as well as for pegging, which is anal penetration with a strap-on.

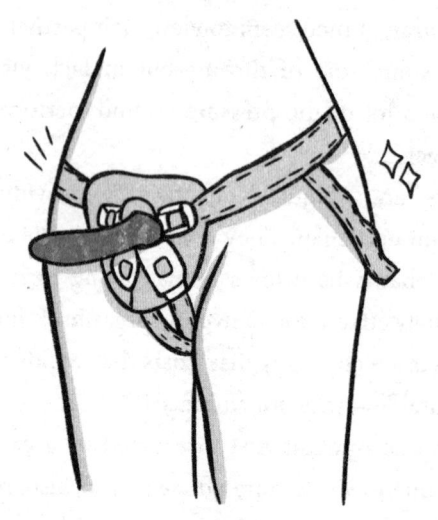

Strap-ons are also sometimes used by people with penises who experience erectile dysfunction. However, anyone can use a strap-on—it's a pleasure product that allows a lot of control and exploration around the experience of penetrative sex.

How do you use a butt plug? – *Shalaka*

A butt plug is a toy that can be inserted into the anus and then stays there while you play. It's meant to provide pleasurable pressure simply while it stays in place—there's no thrusting required. It has a tapered tip for easier insertion, and a stem with a flared base for easy removal. While classic butt plugs are non-motorized, vibrating butt plugs are also available. The flared base or handle is especially important for anal toys, as a toy without one could go too far inside, and become difficult to retrieve.

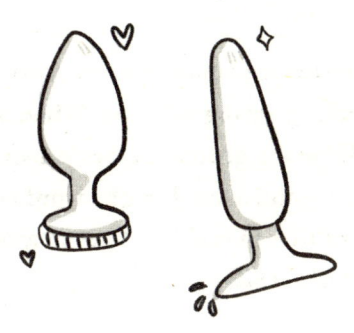

Butt plugs are a gender-neutral toy, and can be a great starting point if anal stimulation is something you're interested in exploring, whether solo or with a partner. If not, that's cool too—there's no pressure to try anything you don't feel comfortable with.

It's worth noting that butt plugs come in different sizes—some people use them as 'anal trainers' to sort of gradually prepare the region and ease into the sensation of anal penetration.

Some vulva-owners find it pleasurable to wear a butt plug during penetrative sex for a feeling of added fullness and stimulation.

No matter your gender, you're definitely going to need lube when using a butt plug, since the anus does not self-lubricate.

If you're new to anal play, the general consensus is that it's best to take things slow. Be gentle and really take your time getting comfortable with it. It's not meant to hurt you.

And again, don't forget: *It's essential to properly clean toys before and after use.*

FANTASIES

My sexual fantasies are sometimes so crazy that I wonder if there's something wrong with me. When masturbating I imagine myself having group sex, or tied up, or having sex in a public place—and even though I would never have the guts to do any of that in real life, I get so aroused thinking about it! Is that ok? – *Sam*

Common Sexual Fantasies

Fantasies are normal, and even the seemingly 'freaky' ones are way more common than we think.

Here are some common categories into which our sexual fantasies may fall into:

Novelty: Fantasies about a new person, place, position or situation. Sometimes these may be novel scenarios that are considered taboo or forbidden.

Multi-partnered sex: Threesomes or group sex, or being watched, or watching others.

Power and control: One might fantasize about being more dominant or more submissive in bed.

Erotic flexibility: Reversing gender roles or sexual-fluidity fantasies are also very common. One may imagine sexual acts that are seemingly inconsistent with how one identifies sexually.

You don't have to act on everything you fantasize about, and if you do want to play out a fantasy, it's really for you and your partner(s) to figure out what you're comfortable or not comfortable with. Informed, mutual, enthusiastic consent is essential.

Q What is role play?

Role play during sex is when partners decide to act out a fantasy or take on the personas of characters in a scene they find exciting—this could include dressing up and costumes, or simply acting out a situation: such as pretending to be doctor and patient or boss and employee or whatever other scenario you both might find erotic.

Many people find roleplay to be a fun way to shed inhibitions in bed and make things extra steamy and sexy—while others may enjoy it as an opportunity to be really goofy and have a laugh together.

FETISHES AND KINKS

Q What is a fetish?

A **fetish** is when you link your sexual arousal to specific objects, materials, or non-genital body parts. For example, one could have a foot or armpit fetish, or a fetish for high heels or stockings.

Whether or not you have a particular fetish, it's often easy enough to see the erotic appeal of common objects and materials that people have fetishes for: leather, latex and velvet, for example, each has its own unique and beautiful appearance and texture that lends itself to a sensory response.

When you think about it, almost anything can fire up the erotic imagination. For instance, even as mundane and everyday an item as fruit can be erotic. Peeling and feeding your lover a lychee; squeezing and sucking a delicious mango—you don't have to have a fruit fetish to be able to see the erotic potential of fruit (although, hey, maybe I *do* have a fruit fetish!).

Q What is a kink?

A **kink** is an unconventional sexual preference or behaviour. But what's considered 'kinky' and 'unconventional' might vary from person to person, given their generation, cultural context and prevalent sexual norms.

For example, our grandparents might consider sex toys or doggy style 'kinky', but these seem fairly vanilla today. BDSM (bondage and discipline, dominance and submission, sadism and masochism), pegging, group sex and cuckolding are examples of sexual preferences currently considered kinks.

While you might think some of your sexual preferences are 'weird' or that no one else has them, the world is actually pretty damn kinky and fetishy behind closed doors. Human sexuality is nuanced and complex. And fun! What really matters is consent.

Common Kinks and Fetishes

BDSM

The acronym 'BDSM' encompasses a range of sexual activities that involve elements of bondage, discipline, sadism and masochism.

An emphasis on informed consent is absolutely central to BDSM because such play often involves varying degrees of pain, physical restraint, domination and submission. Acts may include impact play such as spanking, or rope play, such as having your lover tie you up, or giving and receiving commands—so it is extremely important that both partners share exceptional communication and respect each other's boundaries.

When consensually engaging in acts that could be dangerous, it is necessary to evaluate the risks involved beforehand. Within BDSM terminology, informed consent between individuals is known as SSC (Safe, Sane and Consensual) or RACK (Risk-aware Consensual Kink).

It is also common for partners who engage in BDSM to have a 'safe word' which either partner can say at any point, and the activity would have to stop—this and other such precautions are central to safe and pleasurable BDSM.

The idea is certainly not to harm your partner, but rather to together, consensually, explore each other's arousal, fantasies and pleasure uninhibitedly—many people find aspects of BDSM, power-play and relinquishing control, extremely arousing.

What is femdom? – *Armaan*

Femdom is short for female dominance. Within the kink arena, femdom refers to a dominant feminine partner, typically a dominant woman with a submissive man who wants to obey and please her and follow her commands. The term originates in the BDSM landscape, where a *dominant* describes a partner who takes charge during consensual sex acts involving power, pain or humiliation.

A person can be called a femdom, or an activity can be referred to or described as femdom. It is also a popular genre in porn and erotica. For instance: 'he likes his femdom tying him up' or 'we're curious to try femdom' or 'did you see that femdom video?'

Many people find the idea of femdom especially appealing because it subverts traditional power dynamics—in society, men are expected to be powerful and authoritative while women are expected to be subservient and devoted. In femdom, these gender expectations are reversed.

The domination could be gentle, or more fierce and intense, depending on one another's interests and boundaries. And the roles could be sexual as well as non-sexual—some choose to extend the power dynamics beyond the bedroom as well.

What is a foot fetish? – *Masha*

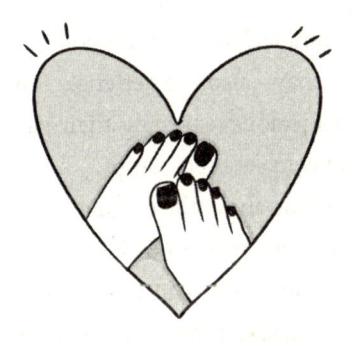

Some people are sexually aroused by feet—this is called a foot fetish. Foot fetishes are extremely common. Many people are drawn to how feet look and feel or to the sense of submissiveness associated with touching someone's feet.

For some people, a foot fetish may extend to enjoying one's partner wearing a particular pair of shoes or, perhaps, preferring their toenails to be painted a certain colour, while for others, just the foot itself may simply function as an object of arousal.

If we're honest, many people enjoy the sensation of their feet being touched—most people like a foot massage, for example—so it can certainly be an erogenous zone that's fun to explore.

What is cuckolding? – *Preet*

Cuckolding is a fetish where a person gets turned on by their partner having sex with someone else.

Why does this turn some people on? Well, it's possible to be aroused by the idea of doing something taboo, or by feelings of sexual jealousy, humiliation or submission.

Some folks may also experience **compersion**—the opposite of sexual jealousy—seeing their partner happy with another person may make them happy.

If you're wondering about the origin of the word 'cuckold', it comes from the cuckoo bird which lays its eggs in other birds' nests such that the birds who had originally made the nests go on to raise chicks that aren't their own. 'Cuckold' was first used in medieval times to refer to the husband of an 'unfaithful' wife who, unaware of his wife's infidelity, would raise children that weren't his own.

In the context of the fetish, the genders of the participants can, of course, vary and the point is that the cuckold actually consents to, enjoys and is aroused by being cuckolded.

As with the practice of any kink or fetish, consent and communication are absolutely central. Clear boundaries are laid out between partners as well as with the third party.

Several kinks and fetishes can seem at odds with our everyday 'morality'. Sometimes we may be turned on by something society tells us we are meant to be upset about—in this case, your partner with another person. *If we acknowledge that the realm of sexual arousal is complex and multifaceted, and if we centre consent, respect and communication as the cornerstones of any sexual exploration, our kinks and fetishes become much more navigable territory.*

PORN

In the internet era, porn has a massive influence on how overarching ideas of what sex is or should be like are being shaped.

Porn is so ubiquitous online that anyone growing up with internet access will likely chance upon porn, whether deliberately or inadvertently, by the time they are ten to twelve years old, if not earlier. And in the absence of comprehensive sex education in schools, as well as a reluctance to share information about sex at home, whether we like it or not, porn is, no doubt, currently serving as the stand-in.

India is one of the world's largest consumers of internet porn. And while the stereotype is that only men watch porn, women watch porn too. In fact, according to data from Porn Hub, at least a quarter of India's users are women.[10]

Q Is porn good or bad? Helpful or harmful?

On the one hand, porn provides the viewer with an experience of arousal or pleasure minus any possibility of infection, accidental pregnancy, or even rejection. Porn certainly has the

---

10 'Despite the Porn Ban, India Is the Third-largest Porn Watcher with 30 Per Cent Female Users', Nandini Yadav, Firstpost, https://www.firstpost.com/tech/news-analysis/despite-porn-ban-india-is-3rd-largest-porn-watcher-with-30-female-users-5721351.html

potential to be a healthy and helpful outlet for our sexual needs and curiosities.

Watching porn can help people feel more comfortable with their sexuality when they see their desires normalized and validated. There are studies that indicate that when porn is watched by couples together, it is often correlated with increased sexual satisfaction and higher levels of intimacy. It can also improve your communication with your partner around sex—like 'ooh, let's try that!' or 'woah! I would not be comfortable doing that!'

But despite some of these benefits, many free porn sites can also be extremely problematic. There's often a lot of ambiguity when it comes to consent—and surely, as a viewer, you do not want to be supporting or participating in the violation of someone's consent. Can you be sure that the act was consensual? Was it consensually filmed? Was the clip consensually shared on the internet?

Also, even when it's a professionally shot clip made by a big studio, where consent has been explicitly given by the actors, the stereotypical 'porn star' aesthetic and imagery remain very much created by and for the straight white male gaze, much like the dominant aesthetic of movies, magazines, music videos and most forms of mainstream international pop culture over the last many decades. The misogyny and violence, the hyper-idealized body types (big dick, big boobs, no body hair), the fetishization of certain races, ages and identities—all of this can exacerbate body-image issues, reiterate regressive gender roles and stereotypes, and provide a very narrow and often unrealistic purview of sex and desire.

You see this even in the way that clips are titled and categorized on mainstream porn sites—it all too often takes the focus away from people experiencing pleasure and reduces them to their gender, size, age, race or body type, phrased in ever-more shocking, violent, 'clickable' ways.

So, how can we shape our relationship with internet porn to ensure that if we do watch it, it influences healthier, more positive sexual experiences, instead of gender-unequal and violent ones?

Several indie adult filmmakers—many of whom are women and queer folk—are already trying to provide a solution to that conundrum by creating 'ethical' porn.

Q What is ethical porn?

It's porn that seeks to mitigate many of the issues with mainstream porn. There's a focus on consent, on more gender-equal and diverse representations of sexuality and pleasure, and on safer sexual practices. Diversity is represented respectfully and authentically rather than in crude, disrespectful ways that reiterate damaging societal prejudices and stereotypes.

The vision is also to create a safe and professional work environment for performers—all performers are necessarily 18+, their health and rights are protected, they're paid equitably, they have a say in who they want to work with and what scenes they are comfortable carrying out.

Ethical porn seeks to produce porn ethically, as well as to portray sex as an emotionally and physically nuanced experience of pleasure, intimacy and discovery, for people of all genders and sexual orientations.

I interviewed Erika Lust, widely considered a pioneer of ethical porn, as well as celebrated indie porn performer Kali Sudhra, about their work. The video is viewable on my Instagram and YouTube—you might enjoy that conversation if you'd like to learn more about ethical porn.

What especially stood out for me from that conversation was the learning that, as a viewer, you have the ability to help shape the porn industry so that everything from casting and production to distribution and the types of situations that are depicted are ethical. How? By being discerning about what we consume, and being willing to pay for it.

If you enjoy watching porn, learn which production companies are driven by ethics. Look for ethical porn and watch only porn that you know is ethical. And understand that for porn to be made professionally and ethically, actors and filmmakers need to get paid equitably. Pay for ethical porn just the same way you'd pay for any other product you enjoy consuming ethically.

If you're wondering where to watch ethical porn, SexSchoolHub.com, and MakeLoveNotPorn.tv are two great places to start. Erika Lust's Xconfessions.com is also fun—here people from all over the world submit descriptions of their sexual fantasies anonymously, and these are turned into erotic short films each month.

There are also several other sites that feature only ethical porn. Once you start looking for it, it's not that hard to find. So, if you do like to watch porn, think about what you choose to watch. Stop watching porn that might be non-consensually or exploitatively made. There's better porn out there already—you just have to make the right choice.

If you'd like to think more critically about porn, its history and its place in our lives, particularly in the Indian context, I highly recommend reading *Cyber Sexy: Rethinking Pornography* by Richa Kaul Padte.

Q Is porn addiction real?

I fear I am addicted to porn. I need to watch it every day. I sometimes think it's not possible for me to experience sexual pleasure without watching porn. What do I do?
– *Yashraj*

I feel really bad about watching porn but I can't stop myself from watching it. I try to stop myself from watching more than once a week but every time I do watch, I find myself choosing more intense or violent clips. Even though I enjoy it while watching, I feel I am doing something really shameful, and then I feel bad about myself. – *Emran*

I get dozens of messages, mainly from men, telling me that they are scared of their relationship with porn; that they feel a lack of control over what and how much they watch; that they find themselves escalating to more and more intense genres, or that their porn consumption interferes with their daily life and their relationships with real people.

Research on 'porn addiction' is still sort of limited and ongoing, and the term is debated quite a lot, with some preferring the term 'compulsive sexual behaviour' over 'addiction'.

It's worth noting that some people who don't actually watch very much porn may also feel excessively guilty about their porn consumption, even if minimal, because they've internalized the messaging that watching porn is always and inherently terribly 'bad' or 'wrong'. If you feel bad about doing something, doing it is likely to make you feel guilty or ashamed.

However, even people who don't feel bad about consuming porn per se often write in saying that after years of frequent porn consumption, they don't enjoy the sort of 'hold' porn seems to have over their experiences of sexual pleasure.

It seems reasonable to consider the fact that internet porn provides unlimited access to unlimited new clips, which means that if you enjoy watching porn, both novelty and sexual stimulus—two rather powerful and exciting things—are available to you indefinitely, in a way that was never possible back when there was no internet.

The very nature of most internet media, in fact, is to make it difficult to stop watching. Whether it's a movie streaming platform or even a news site, you have so many options for what to watch, and you're constantly offered more and more content to consume. Content will often even auto play—they want you to stay on there for as long as possible.

As websites and apps get better at recognizing your tastes and preferences from the videos you choose to watch, they show you more and more of whatever they think will keep you there.

In this way, even social media has a highly 'addictive' quality to it. We've all been there—wondering how we've been stuck scrolling for two hours, and realizing we're never getting that time back.

Another thing that's important to consider is that when an adult with a fully developed brain and pre-existing sexual experience accesses porn, they might look for clips that match their pre-existing ideas and fantasies around sex—and porn might even be a fun and healthy outlet for that sexual energy. You already have some idea of what a healthy sexual relationship looks like, you kind of already know what turns you on, and you might seek that out in porn.

But in the internet age, people are accessing porn, whether deliberately or accidentally, as young as nine or ten years old, or even younger, most often with no prior reference point or understanding of sex. The perspectives of a person that young are much more susceptible to being shaped by the imagery or influences they are exposed to.

Because of its sheer ubiquity, porn might also inordinately impact our ideas around what a desirable body should look like, and which sexual acts are pleasurable—even though too often in mainstream porn the acts are unrealistically extreme, violent and misogynistic.

Some people may even find that habitual porn use makes them more likely to see porn as a necessary condition for arousal—it can become difficult to feel aroused with a real person or even difficult to climax without porn.

Feeling like you have no control over what or how much porn you watch can lead to feelings of fear and anxiety, as can most behaviours over which you begin to feel a lack of control.

If you find yourself in a situation where your relationship with porn seems like a problem to you, it is certainly worth thinking about. If it's impacting your mental health or getting in the way of your ability to fulfil your work, school, or family commitments, for example, maybe it's time to cut back?

Unfortunately, masturbation and porn often get bucketed together—but it's worth remembering that it is possible to enjoy self-pleasure without porn. Using your imagination can be a wonderful thing to do instead.

Q What shapes our sexual and romantic aspirations?

Zooming out a little, it's worth thinking about the dominant forces that shape our sexual and romantic preferences and aspirations. Not just in bed, but even in terms of what we envision the 'ideal relationship' or 'ideal sexual encounter' to be.

Mainstream porn and the glorification of weddings are among the most pervasive pop cultural imagery we receive, and we should be aware of their impact. Marriage is so central to the way society is structured, and mainstream porn is so central to the way the internet is structured, that even if you'd rather not encounter them, they're likely to find you!

Unsurprisingly, these forces have an enormous influence on what many of us think we must aspire to in our relationships and our sexual lives. And too often they collapse rather than expand our sexual and romantic imagination.

Also, while people of all genders are subject to these forces, there is a gendered aspect to it too, where marriage can feel particularly inescapable for women, and porn can feel particularly inescapable for men. Plus, in their most mainstream formats, marriage and porn too often exclude queer people.

Let your imagination remind you of the infinite possibilities that lie beyond these two boxes! For starters: relationship structures outside of compulsory endogamous opposite-sex monogamy only, and sex that involves connection, care, vulnerability, kindness, trust, genuine affection, attention and intimacy.

Personally, I don't intend to get married, and I don't watch mainstream porn. I'm not saying my choices are for everyone, but I do think it's worth at least considering that it is possible to have a meaningful and fulfilling sexual and romantic life without these.

Unfortunately, many people don't really have a choice. Marriage is too often an inevitability rather than a choice, that it can be very near impossible to opt out of for many. And mainstream porn is so omnipresent on the internet that you often don't even have to search for it; you will stumble upon it, most likely before you've had the opportunity to develop your own ideas about sex.

I think this stuff is important to be aware of, so you can allow yourself the possibility to imagine something different too.

Relationships

Navigating Sexuality Together

TALKING TO YOUR FAMILY ABOUT SEX

I wish I could talk to my parents about sex. I'm 25 years old and I live with my parents, and even though I work and support myself, I can't bring anyone over to the house. It would be so much easier to have safer sexual experiences, access contraception, go to the gynac, if I could just talk to my parents about it instead of having to find ways to do all of this secretly. – *Somaya*

How do we talk to our kids about sex? We don't want to be the type of parents who our kids are too afraid to turn to when they have a problem–but we have no idea where to even begin. We have a 10-year-old and a 12-year-old and we can sense that they are curious about sex and the body, given whatever they may have seen in movies or found out about with their friends. How do we have a conversation with them? Is it a one-time conversation? How should we go about it? – *Rahila* and *Sid*

In a perfect world, families would be able to talk about sex.

Instead of shying away from the subject or punishing children for asking questions, parents would proactively talk to their kids about sexuality, sexual health and the body, and kids would be able to ask their parents whatever questions might arise as they grow up, knowing they will receive honest, judgement-free answers. Sadly that's rarely the case.

In fact, one of the most frequent questions I get in my DMs every time I post a new video is: do your parents know about your channel? Or: are your parents okay with the fact that you talk about sex?

Of course they know about my channel—it's on the internet—and I've got to admit, I really lucked out in the parents department—they've long been my greatest supporters.

In many ways, I can talk about all the things I talk about *because* of them—they made sure home felt like a safe space where we could ask about anything, and would provide straightforward, scientifically accurate answers to our questions—even about sex and the body.

They're still always the first people I turn to when I have any sort of health or relationship question or problem or need advice.

But many people *never* talk to their families about sex. There's so much discomfort and shame around these subjects that these conversations just don't happen.

Or if they do happen, there tends to be this idea that the conversation only has to be had once—'the talk'—where parents hurriedly and awkwardly bring it up with teenage kids to scare the living daylights out of them and tell them sex is evil. And then never talk about it again.

Have you talked to your parents about sex? If you're a parent, have you talked to your kids about sex? If you have, how did you approach it and how did it go? What do you think we could do to make these conversations feel safer, more comfortable and less awkward?

Ideally, parents should talk to their kids about sex, sexuality, sexual health and the body not just once, but rather all through their upbringing, in age-appropriate, judgement-free ways. It is never too early to start. And it's not a one-time conversation.

For example, parents should teach toddlers the scientifically accurate names for their genitals, just like we teach them the names of all other body parts. If we teach kids words like nose and stomach and knee and ankle so that they can learn about their bodies, then why do we teach them euphemisms for their genitals—or else not teach them about the genitals at all? After all, these are also just parts of the body.

Penis, scrotum, vulva, vagina, etc., are just the scientifically accurate names for those parts of our bodies. By using made-up words for them, or by refusing to name them, we help ingrain a sense of shame in a child about their own body, making it seem like there's something bad, embarrassing or unspeakable about these body parts.

Think about some of the euphemisms you may have been taught as a kid as names for genitals. Along with silly or funny-sounding words like 'nunu' and 'chuchu', many parents even tell their little children that the name for their genitals is 'shame-shame'. Think about how that's going to impact a young person's perspective on their body and sexuality. Wouldn't it be great if we could get comfortable simply using anatomically accurate words, just as we teach them the names of all other body parts?

As babies grow into little people with the ability to say yes and no, parents can begin to inculcate an intuitive understanding of consent. This becomes more and more important as a child starts interacting with others, going to playschool and making friends.

We tend to often raise kids without actually allowing them any autonomy or agency—with a 'you will do as I say' approach. But this sends the message that their consent doesn't matter. It's helpful to explain to children why you're setting a certain rule or boundary, why you're encouraging or discouraging a certain activity or behaviour, and how it benefits their well-being, instead of simply using a 'because I said so' approach.

And parents should answer the inevitable questions that will arise about where babies come from accurately. Explaining the science in a simple and age-appropriate way, such as with a basic diagram of sperm and egg, and of a foetus developing in the womb—instead of making up a story—is arguably the better approach. As the child grows older and more mature, you can elaborate on the explanation as and when the topic comes up.

As children approach their preteen years, parents can discuss the natural changes in the body that will take place during puberty, including menstruation. Personally, I think everything should be explained to kids of all genders, rather than having separate 'talks with girls' and 'talks with boys'.

Ideally, parents of adolescents should also discuss portrayals of sex and sexuality in the media before their kids end up stumbling upon porn without any context to turn to.

In the internet era, porn is so omnipresent that if you have a child and internet access, the likelihood of the child accessing porn, whether deliberately or inadvertently, whether by themselves or through a peer, is extremely high.

It's therefore important that we equip young people with an understanding of consent; of the fact that studio-produced porn is performed by professional actors; that it's a form of media intended for adult entertainment; that our bodies don't all look like mainstream porn bodies; and that the violence and misogyny present in a lot of mainstream porn is extremely problematic. Cultivating the critical thinking skills to be discerning about media and porn portrayals of sex, enables young people to develop more informed, positive and healthy attitudes to sexuality and the body.

Over the teenage years, parents also ought to explain the risks that come with sex, including STIs and accidental pregnancy, as well as the basics of safer sex and contraception, so that their kids are able to make safer, smarter choices when they begin to navigate relationships of their own.

Contrary to what some seem to fear, talking to your kids about sex isn't going to make them rush out recklessly to have sex ASAP. Quite the opposite, in fact. Research tells us that kids and teens who are able to talk with their parents and caregivers about sex and relationships are more likely to delay having sex, less likely to take risks with their or another person's health and safety, as well as have better mental health.

And it really isn't just a single conversation—it needs to be an ongoing one. These conversations can start when the child is a toddler and progress all the way through adulthood.

But, sadly, many families *never* talk openly and honestly about sex.

So if you're a teenager or a young adult and your parents have never talked to you about sex, the good news is that, even though I said it's never too early to start, it's never too late to start either.

And since, perhaps because of their own upbringing or baggage or conditioning, your parents haven't been able to approach the subject with you, you may want to consider being the one to initiate the conversation.

Talking with your parents about sex can feel super scary—but again, here, too, don't think of it as one big talk about everything all at once.

It can be easier to try to incorporate conversations about sexuality, sexual health and the body in little ways, so they slowly become a topic that is up for discussion without stigma.

Starting the conversation the first time can be the hardest part. But it usually gets easier and easier over time.

Here are some tips to help you out:

You can try using a relevant article or show you've watched—such as *Sex Education* on Netflix—or any of the videos on my handles, as a springboard to start talking about sex more generally. Then you can work your way up to the stuff that's more personal to you.

Think of questions you want to ask. You could ask them about what their parents taught them about sex, or about what it feels like to be in love, or about their thoughts on contraception—or whatever else you'd like to discuss with them.

Tell them why you're asking. Explain to them that you think it would be helpful to be able to talk openly about these things with them instead of having to look for information elsewhere.

Maybe you also want to get a sense of what they expect from you? Or maybe you want their help making a decision. Explaining why you want to talk about stuff will perhaps help them better understand where you are coming from and prevent them from making assumptions.

If you feel more comfortable approaching the subject by writing them a note or sending an email or text message, you can do that instead. It doesn't matter *how* you talk—just talk.

If it feels super awkward to talk to your parents about sex, you can perhaps initiate the conversation by first acknowledging the awkwardness. You could perhaps say something like: 'This feels awkward for me to talk about, and maybe it feels awkward for you too, but I think it's important for us to be able to discuss this stuff.' Sometimes, acknowledging the discomfort can help in working through it.

But what if you really just *cannot* talk to your parents or family about sex?

Unfortunately, some people cannot seem to get over their discomfort around sex, and may even threaten or punish their kids for bringing it up. If you feel that asking questions about sex could in any way put you in danger, don't do it. Also, some people may not have access to their parents. In these cases, they could talk to a kind, respectful and knowledgeable adult family member or caregiver they trust.

Hopefully, even by just thinking about this stuff, we can help end the cycle of perpetuating shame, stigma, and misinformation around sexuality and the body, instead of passing it on to the next generation. So that even if your parents weren't able to talk to you about sex in a healthy way, you will be able to do so with your children, should you choose to have any. At least that's my hope.

And to any parent reading this, please listen to your children with an open mind and an open heart. Even if you don't always agree with them.

Q What does a healthy relationship look like?

A healthy relationship is one in which you feel cared for and respected; where you trust one another, and you feel free, not stifled; one in which you are able to be true to yourself, *where you don't have to pretend*. And in a healthy relationship, you should never have to fear for your well-being or safety.

Looking back, I started out pretty terrible at relationships. I thought that a 'good' relationship had no place for conflict. I would hide any uncomfortable feelings—disappointment, anger, sadness—till I could no longer pretend, and that resulted in more than one absolutely catastrophic break-up, as well as a withering away of a handful of friendships.

I now realize that in a healthy relationship, you should be able to both love someone and disagree with them. Relationships take work, and in a healthy relationship, both people put in an effort to work through things together—but also allow each other space for differences. It is possible to be deeply empathetic and compassionate and patient with one another, to be a great team, while still always feeling whole yourself. To be good at relationships is to be good at listening, forgiving and, sometimes, even letting go if that's what's best for one or either of you.

A healthy relationship is honest, not manipulative; loving, without being all-consuming. Both parties deserve to feel equal in decision-making. A healthy relationship also holds space for the other things that may be important to each person: careers, friendships, hobbies.

A healthy relationship is one in which both people, at their cores, feel good about being with each other, and are together because they genuinely want to be, not just out of a sense of obligation to each other, family or society.

How important is sex to a relationship? Does the quality of the sex and the quality of a relationship go hand in hand? I'm married and I love my husband as a person, but the sex is far from satisfying, as he hardly ever makes time

for it and, when he does, he doesn't seem to know what he's doing. I'm wondering whether that will impact our relationship long term. Like, is this really it? Do I resign myself to a lifetime of infrequent and unsatisfying sex? Should I leave him? Can he become a better lover? I don't know what to do. – *Cherie*

Over time I've come to understand that some people are just very good at sex like some people are very good at swimming or cycling or dancing. Just because the sex is good doesn't mean that you two are meant to be. And on the flipside—just because the sex isn't sizzling, it doesn't mean it can't get better.

And this was news to me. For the longest time, I mistakenly assumed that my pleasure in bed was contingent on my partner's abilities. I hadn't considered that it could be contingent on my own.

By becoming an expert at your own pleasure, the sex you're having often becomes considerably more fun. Once you really understand your own pleasure, you can initiate positions that you know will work for you, and communicate with your partner in great detail about what you enjoy. You can also add a toy to the mix—it can help you navigate your own pleasure extremely effectively and also ease some of the pressure on your partner to 'perform'.

But it's hard to make any of these changes if you and your partner aren't able to talk about sex. So work towards getting comfortable talking to each other about the sex you're having. What feels good, what doesn't, what are your curiosities, and what are your boundaries. It can be quite a fun exercise to go over a list of sexual acts together and play 'yes, no, maybe,' to indicate to each other, in a pressure-free way, what might be exciting to explore, and what either of you are definitely not into.

It's also very common for couples to have variations in libido—one person may want sex more often than the other, for example. And that's okay. It can help to identify what you want from sex. Is it the physical release—an orgasm? Masturbating can help take care of that too. Is it a sense of closeness and intimacy? Perhaps cuddling and making eye contact and just holding each other can provide that. If one person isn't quite as sexual as the other, it isn't anyone's fault. And finding ways to do activities other than intercourse—either together or solo—that provide a sense of closeness and pleasure can actually even expand your ideas of intimacy.

Scheduling sex—even though that might not sound so sexy—can be another rather useful approach, especially if you and your partner live together and have been together a long time. Because, among the long list of daily commitments people have—running a home, work, kids, etc.—sex can easily be relegated to the bottom.

People who don't live together kind of have to schedule dates and sex in any case—and you'd think that wouldn't be a problem when you live with someone—but, ironically, when you can theoretically do something anytime, it's the easiest to put off for later. Scheduling sex can even serve as a form of foreplay—it can give you both something to look forward to, to build anticipation towards. Try it if it sounds like it may work for you.

I do think that sexual compatibility and general compatibility are not one and the same. You could be having amazing sex with someone who is impossible to live with, and you could have a fantastic everyday partnership with someone who isn't the best sex you've ever had—of course, it would be great to have both, and I do think it's something partners can together work towards. But I think it's worth keeping in mind that a successful long-term relationship—both on the sexual front and on the general front—is rarely the result of magic and, more often, takes deliberate and sustained work.

Ultimately, only you can decide whether the sex is a dealbreaker or whether you like being with your partner enough to work through this together.

Toxic Masculinity

The dumbest, most harmful sh*t is associated with masculinity at times—downright awful stuff like refusing to wear a condom, harassing women, or getting into a physical fight are considered 'masculine' and often glorified. I don't want to be that type of 'man'. How can I do better? Also, it can often seem like many women are so traumatized by their past interactions with men that it's very hard to even get a date on a dating app or win over their trust at the start of a relationship. What can I do to make it clear that I'm not like that? – *Anirudh*

It's so profoundly disappointing that, globally, masculinity still, in many ways, remains defined by a predisposition for violence and the degradation of women. In a patriarchal society, men are raised to believe they should 'protect' the 'honour' of the women in their family, while feeling free to objectify and/or harm other women. Men have been actively discouraged from seeing or communicating with women as equals for so long that the idea that masculine is superior and feminine is inferior has been internalized to the point that it simply seems like the natural order of the world. In fact, most cishet upper-caste men have internalized the degradation of anyone who is not cishet male and upper-caste.

And we have got to do something about it.

Rape, honour killings, acid attacks, domestic violence and sexual harassment, both offline and online—these are such an everyday occurrence that the headlines don't even surprise us anymore. And all too often these acts are excused because of how attached we are to this toxic brand of masculinity. How easily we instead blame the victims: 'boys will be boys', 'she was asking for it'.

How are we okay with this?

The situation is even worse for women and queer people from communities which have been historically discriminated against. The misogyny becomes coupled with casteism, communalism, ableism, racism, homophobia and transphobia.

The reality is that virtually ALL women have experienced some degree of sexual violence or harassment perpetrated by a man in real life or online, or both. So while men like to claim that it's not all men, it is way too many men. Of course, that leaves us exhausted and weary, and unable to easily trust men.

And toxic masculinity does not just actively harm women and minorities. It harms men too.

By ending rape culture, by dismantling patriarchal systems that perpetuate violence and inequality, men wouldn't be doing some sort of favour to anyone. They would be acting in their own best interest.

Surely men would benefit from being able to express themselves in ways other than just strength, anger and violence. Surely men would like to be able to be vulnerable, to express emotion, without shame. Surely more men would enjoy being able to walk away from the pressure to pursue the accrual of wealth and property as the sole purpose of their life's work. Surely men would like to be able to ask for help and to associate their self-worth with something other than just their masculinity. But who's standing in the way of them being able to do all this cool stuff? Ideas of masculinity. Constructed by ... wait for it—men!

An equal world isn't about less rights for men and more rights for others; it's a world where gender, caste, religion, sexual orientation and all the rest ceases to be a cause for discrimination and violence. It's a world where we would all be better off—men too, in fact, perhaps men most of all—because toxic masculinity is in fact not a fun trap to be stuck in at all, as Anirudh, who sent in the question, admits.

But the burden of this labour of unlearning—of challenging the dominant conditioning, of dismantling toxic masculinity—shouldn't have to be carried out solely by women and queer people. Men, you need to hold each other accountable; hold each other to a higher standard; remind each other that you are capable of better; and actively reject what patriarchy has taught you. The only way women who don't know you will be able to more easily believe that you are a safe, kind and respectful person, Anirudh, is if we can more easily believe that about all men.

In the meantime, being mindful of this in your interactions with women is a start. Understand where the hesitation comes from. Be kind and respectful, even when you don't get the response you might have been hoping for. It can be very refreshing to meet a man who is never creepy or pushy or entitled, who is self-aware and understands boundaries, and who is just as happy to be your friend if sex isn't on the cards.

Non-monogamy

What exactly is polyamory? How is it different from cheating? – *Parth*

Ethical non-monogamy and **polyamory** refer to relationship structures where people may have more than one partner, with the consent of everyone involved. It is different from cheating for this very reason—there is no deception—because boundaries and expectations have been established in advance.

It is also different from historical/cultural/religious practices like polygamy—where a man would have multiple wives; or polyandry—where a woman would have multiple husbands, as it does not have an inherently gendered aspect to who can have the multiple partners. Plus, it is not a socially imposed norm but rather a matter of personal choice. Ethical non-monogamy depends on the willing participation of all parties.

When a couple is in a monogamous relationship, the expectation between the two people is that they will each be the other's only partner. So if you're in a monogamous relationship and you seek a sexual or romantic interaction with someone else, it can feel like a massive betrayal to your partner because the expectation was monogamy.

But monogamy isn't for everyone.

There are more and more people exploring ethical non-monogamy because the idea of a monogamous marriage (society's default setting for how relationships are structured)—that you have to be everything for each other, forever—can feel pretty stifling and unrealistic to many.

Ethical non-monogamy or polyamory can take a variety of forms. Some people have a primary partner whom they love and live with, for example, and with whom rules and boundaries are established around whether and how either or both parties can interact with others in a sexual or romantic capacity. Some poly folks may have more than one primary partner. And multiple people who are sexually and/or romantically involved with one another together could form a 'polycule'.

That is not to say that in contrast to the often-dissatisfying experience of monogamy, non-monogamy is all bubblegum and roses. Non-monogamy has its own challenges too.

For example, people in ethically non-monogamous relationship structures may experience feelings of jealousy, hurt or insecurity despite having consented to their partner being able to see other people, and despite the fact that they too are seeing other people. These are feelings to be worked through together.

Non-monogamy isn't for everyone either, and it can be complicated to navigate given how deeply social norms still remain oriented around monogamy globally. But it does seem to provide a vision of greater freedom and autonomy that an ever-growing number of people find appealing.

Confused about Your Sexuality?

I'm confused about my sexual orientation. I thought I was straight, and I've had boyfriends in the past, but more recently I feel like I'm also strongly attracted to women. Am I bisexual? Am I a lesbian? I've never actually had a relationship or a sexual experience with a woman so does that mean I'm still technically straight until I have one? How do I know how I identify sexually? – *Vidhi*

While some people feel like they've always innately identified a certain way, for many of us, it's an ongoing process of self-discovery.

Most aspects of the human experience involve a complex interaction of our biology, our psychology and the social/cultural world around us, making it impossible to totally distinguish each from the other or draw a definitive causal relationship around what exactly determines something like our sexuality.

Most of us inherit the idea that heterosexuality or opposite-sex attraction is the default. So many of us may find ourselves having to unpack our own identity from that internalized idea of **'compulsory heterosexuality'**. And that can be an ongoing process.

In addition to 'heterosexual', 'cis man' or 'cis woman', which is what it can still feel like society just assumes us to all be, there are lots of different labels out there for sexual orientation and gender identity—gay, lesbian, bisexual, pansexual, asexual, trans, nonbinary, agender, genderqueer. I have described these terms in the glossary at the start of the book. It can be helpful to familiarize yourself with them in case any of them help you describe yourself—but there's also no pressure to identify with just one or any of them.

You may also find that how you feel sexually and who you're attracted to can evolve over time as you get to know yourself better. And that's fine too!

Your understanding of your sexuality can expand as you discover parts of yourself you hadn't yet become acquainted with. This can happen as you become better able to distinguish between the social and cultural expectations and conditioning you've internalized, and your own feelings and sense of self—and whether or not, or how much, the two overlap.

It's okay to feel confused or unsure of how you identify, and it's okay if a label that once felt true to you no longer encompasses how you feel. Embrace your own path of self-discovery.

You don't have to have had a sexual or romantic relationship with someone of the same gender, or present yourself in a particular way in order to establish that you're queer. *Your sexual orientation and gender identity are yours to understand and express on your own terms, they require no external 'qualifications' or validation.*

Sadly, society can make it feel like our bodies and sexualities are everyone else's business but our own. The truth is, you don't have to prove anything to anyone—in simply seeking to always be true to yourself, you owe no explanations.

Love

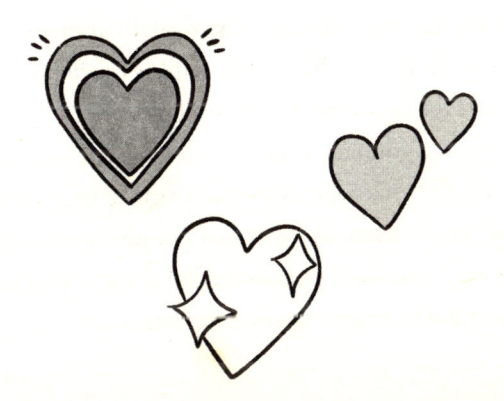

I know this book is about sex, but how can we not also talk about love? Our physical and emotional well-being are deeply connected—and I want to acknowledge and honour this connection.

I think it really behoves us to unburden love from the trappings of the dominant ideas of strictly cishet monogamous romance that have so weighed it down. Ideas of 'the one', of a single 'soulmate', while perhaps cute, really don't actually serve us, and they don't even hold much water. And this is not me being a grumpy, bitter, cynical pessimist—quite the opposite. I think of love as one of the greatest joys life has to offer—loving and being loved is perhaps *the* greatest thing about being alive in my opinion.

So why restrict opening up your heart to the wonders of that feeling till you identify said mystical soulmate? Why restrict your capacity for warmth, care, empathy, generosity, and a willingness to listen as if large-heartedness is a thing to be rationed? Are we not all, in fact, inherently worthy of being treated by one another as respectable and loveable and valuable by virtue of our shared humanity? Surely you do not have to be planning on marriage and babies with someone in order for them to deserve to be treated with warmth, kindness and respect, and for you to be worthy of theirs.

When I was younger, I used to conflate sex and love, and I used to idealize marriage. But now I realize that sex and love do not always overlap, and that just because someone is good at one doesn't necessarily mean they're going to be good at the other. And that marriage need not feature at all.

Contrary to the message society tries to hammer in, a romantic relationship or marriage is not the only context within which love can be legitimately explored. Love can be friendship; love can be living together; it can be looking after yourself. Love does not have to last forever to be valuable. Love can be non-monogamous; it can simply be sharing or creating something special. Honestly, love can be your whole entire attitude to life.

And I believe it's something you have to practice. We're not just magically good at love when we need to be. It's something you have to work at to get better at. Love isn't static and it isn't automatic. The most reliable way to get better at love, all kinds of love, is simply by loving. Love every day. Love as much as you can.

Afterword

Now that you have read *The Sex Book* and are equipped with this basic but fairly comprehensive information about sex, relationships and the body, I hope that you feel empowered to embark on the adventure that is navigating the terrain of your own sexuality in the most joyful, safe and pleasurable ways possible.

I hope you're now inspired to think about who you are sexually, what gives you pleasure, what you're looking for in a relationship, a friendship, or in a lover, as well as what kind of friend or partner or lover you want to be—whether to yourself or to someone you desire or care for.

If you're already sexually active, look back on the sexual experiences that stand out for the exuberance and joy they brought you, as well as the ones that may have seemed unfulfilling for whatever reason. What made the really good experiences so good, and what could either of you have done differently to make the not-so-good experiences better?

If you're not yet sexually active, know that there's no hurry. Take your time. If you never intend on being sexually active, that's completely fine too. Reflect on your experiences and preferences, think about what you want and what you don't want. What you like, what you don't like. What you're curious about, what your boundaries are.

Wherever you are in your own sexual journey, I hope you'll be inspired to understand and explore your own body, to cultivate a self-pleasure practice, if you haven't already, if that's something that sounds like it might be fun to you. Take the time to figure out what arouses you, what makes you feel seen, what makes you feel safe, what makes your heart dance.

I hope you'll be inspired to set out on your very own joyful journey of sexual self-discovery.

As I said at the beginning of this book, sex has long been constructed as if it is necessarily heterosexual, and gender has long been constructed as if it is necessarily binary. The framework most of us inherit in terms of how sex is imagined is as if sex is necessarily penis-in-vagina penetration. Men are the necessary predators and women only reluctant and/or dutiful participants in the context of a marital relationship, or else the necessary gatekeepers, forbidden from seeking or expressing their own desire or pleasure. Sex is also deeply associated with shame—but, ironically, people are shamed both for having sex as well as for not wanting sex.

I'd like to see us totally reframe how we see sex such that we eliminate the shame, and our vision enables greater equality: centering consent, enabling the agency and autonomy of women and queer people, eliminating discrimination on the basis of sexual orientation and gender identity, recognizing and making more space for asexuality—that some people may not be driven by sex at all—and dismantling the violence inherent in our construction of masculinity.

I'd like us to imagine a world where all sexual experiences are consensual, safe and pleasurable—for everyone, of all genders and sexual orientations.

FURTHER READING

If you liked reading this book and are eager to learn more, here are five books that I love that I think you might enjoy too!

Come As You Are, Emily Nagoski

Becoming Cliterate, Laurie Mintz

Beyond The Gender Binary, Alok Vaid-Menon

The Tragedy of Heterosexuality, Jane Ward

Cyber Sexy: Rethinking Pornography, Richa Kaul Padte

Acknowledgements

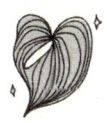

It would be so much harder to do the work I do—talking about sex publicly—if my family weren't my biggest supporters. Arjun, Ritu, Buddha, Leena, Debbie, Aditya, Shruti, Nani, and my darling Little Bear—thank you for always sharing my conviction in the fact that it is important to talk about this stuff. In so many ways, each of you has shaped who I am and how I see the world.

Mom and Papa, thank you for being the coolest, funnest, most loving and inspired people and parents. Thank you for always being unapologetically yourselves. I've learned from the best!

Little Bear, I love that you celebrate me every day. Thank you for telling me to put my work on social media when you did, and for championing me every step of the way. Seeing as you've been stuck with me for as long as I've been a sex educator, one of my greatest joys is hearing how deftly you can explain the anatomy of the vulva.

Thank you to Diya Kar, my delightful editor, for getting me to write this book, and for holding my hand through the process. Two years ago, the idea of writing A WHOLE BOOK seemed so impossibly daunting—yet here we are. What a treat that I got to do this with you; it couldn't have been anyone else.

Thank you to Ipsita Divedi, powerhouse feminist illustrator, sexuality education enthusiast, and totally adorable human being, for your beautiful drawings.

Thank you to Paloma Dutta, Amit Malhotra, Akriti Tyagi, Amrita Mukerji, Poulomi Chatterjee, Sohela Singh, Shabnam Srivastava, Rahul Dixit, Ananth Padmanabhan and everyone at HarperCollins India who has helped make this book a reality.

Thank you to Dr Nozer Sheriar for always being willing to answer my questions about sexual and reproductive health and rights in India. I am tremendously grateful for your generosity, care and guidance.

Thank you to Anne Philpott, Arushi Singh and all the wonderful pleasure fellows at The Pleasure Project for so wholeheartedly sharing knowledge and resources, and for the passion with which you advocate for pleasure-inclusive sexual health communications. I've brought much of what I learnt during my Pleasure Fellowship to this book.

And. Thank. YOU. Most of all. YOU. For watching, listening to, and/or reading the sex-ed that I create. None of this would be possible without you. I'm so very grateful we are on this journey together.

About the Author

Leeza Mangaldas is India's foremost sex education content creator. She established her now immensely popular sex-ed platforms on YouTube and Instagram in 2017 as a passion project, alongside her work as a freelance journalist and TV presenter, hoping to help normalize conversations around sexuality, sexual health, gender and the body. Her videos now reach millions of people in India and around the world, daily. She also hosts 'The Sex Podcast', a Spotify exclusive, in Hindi. She is a UN Women Ally, as well as a recipient of The Pleasure Project Fellowship.

She has won several awards for her work, including Sexual Health Influencer of the Year 2021–22 at the *Cosmopolitan* India Blogger Awards, and has featured on *GQ*'s list of Most Influential Young Indians in 2021 and 2022.

Leeza studied English literature and visual art at Columbia University with a focus on gender and sexuality. She lives in Goa with her dog, Mouse. This is her first book.